Workbook for

Fundamental Concepts and Skills for the Patient Care Technician

Workbook for

Fundamental Concepts and Skills for the Patient Care Technician

Second Edition

Kimberly Townsend Little, PhD, RN, CNE
Chair, MSN Programs
School of Nursing
Liberty University
Lynchburg, Virginia

ELSEVIER

Elsevier
3251 Riverport Lane
St. Louis, Missouri 63043

Workbook for Fundamental Concepts and Skills for the Patient
Care Technician, Second Edition   ISBN: 978-0-323-83128-4

Previous editions copyrighted 2018.

Content Strategist: Sonya Seigafuse
Content Development Specialist: Andrae Akeh
Publishing Services Manager: Deepthi Unni
Project Manager: Sindhuraj Thulasingam
Design Direction: Gopalakrishnan Venkatraman

Printed in India

Last digit is the print number: 9   8   7   6   5   4   3

To The Student

This workbook is written to be used with *Fundamental Concepts and Skills for the Patient Care Technician*, second edition, by Kimberly Little Townsend. Any reference to the "textbook" in this workbook refers to *Fundamental Concepts and Skills for the Patient Care Technician*, second edition.

This workbook is designed to help you apply what you have learned in each chapter. You are encouraged to use this workbook as a study guide. Various types of study questions (matching, fill in the blank, multiple choice, and short answer) and other learning activities are included to help you understand and apply the information in the textbook.

Procedure checklists are provided that correspond with the skills in *Fundamental Concepts and Skills for the Patient Care Technician*, second edition. These checklists are intended to help you become confident and skilled when performing procedures that affect the quality of care you provide.

The answers to the workbook questions are provided as part of the instructor resources. Your instructor will provide the answers as needed.

Patient care technicians are important members of the health care team. Completing the exercises in this workbook and strengthening your study skills will increase your knowledge, skills, and confidence. The goal is to prepare you to provide the best possible care and to help you develop pride in the important work you do.

Study Hints for All Students

Ask questions! There are no bad questions. If you do not know something or are not sure, you need to find out. Other people may be wondering the same thing but may be too shy to ask. The answer could mean life or death to your patient, which certainly is more important than feeling embarrassed about asking a question.

Make use of chapter objectives. At the beginning of each chapter in the textbook are objectives that you should have mastered when you finished studying that chapter. Write these objectives in your notebook, leaving a blank space after each. Fill in the answers as you find them while reading the chapter. Review to make sure your answers are correct and complete, and use these answers when you study for tests. This should also be done for separate course objectives that your instructor has listed in your class syllabus.

Locate and understand key terms. At the beginning of each chapter in the textbook are key terms that you will encounter as you read the chapter. The key terms are in bold font the first time they appear in the chapter.

Get the most from your textbook. When reading each chapter in the textbook, look at the subject headings to learn what each section is about. Read first for the general meaning, then reread parts you did not understand.

It may help to read those parts aloud. Carefully read the information given in each table and study each figure and its caption.

Follow up on difficult concepts. While studying, put difficult concepts into your own words to see if you understand them. Check this understanding with another student or the instructor. Write these in your notebook.

Take useful notes. When taking lecture notes in class, leave a large margin on the left side of each notebook page and write only on right-hand pages, leaving all left-hand pages blank. Look over your lecture notes soon after each class, while your memory is fresh. Fill in missing words, complete sentences and ideas, and underline key phrases, definitions, and concepts. At the top of each page, write the topic of that page. In the left margin, write the key word for that part of your notes. On the opposite left-hand page, write a summary or outline that combines material from both the textbook and the lecture. These can be your study notes for review.

Join or form a study group. Form a study group with some other students so you can help one another. Practice speaking and reading aloud, ask questions about material you are not sure about, and work together to find answers.

Improve your study skills. Good study skills are essential for achieving your goals. Time management, efficient use of study time, and a consistent approach to studying are all beneficial.

Additional Study Hints for Students Who Use English as a Second Language

Find a first-language buddy. ESL students should find a first-language buddy – another student who is a native speaker of English and is willing to answer questions about word meanings, pronunciations, and culture. Maybe your buddy would like to learn about your language and culture. This could help in his or her health care experience as well.

Expand your vocabulary. If you find a nontechnical word you do not know (e.g., *drowsy*), try to guess its meaning from the sentence (e.g., *With electrolyte imbalance, the patient may feel fatigued and drowsy*). If you are not sure of the meaning, or if it seems particularly important, look it up in the dictionary.

Keep a vocabulary notebook. Keep a small alphabetical notebook or address book in which you can write down new nontechnical words you read or hear along with their meanings and pronunciations. Write each word under its initial letter so you can find it easily, as in a dictionary. For words you do not know or for words that have a different meaning in health care, write down how they are used and sound. Look up their meanings in a dictionary or ask your instructor or first-language buddy. Then write the different meanings or usages that you have found in your book, including the health care meaning. Continue to add new words as you discover them. For example:

Primary – Of most importance; main (e.g., *the primary problem or disease*); The first one; elementary (e.g., *primary school*)

Secondary – Of less importance; resulting from another problem or disease (e.g., *a secondary symptom*); The second one (e.g., *secondary school* [*"high school" in the United States*])

Contents

Answerkeys are available online

This page intentionally left blank

Today's Healthcare _____

MATCHING

Directions: Match the key terms on the left with the description on the right.

Key Terms	Description
_____ 1. health *(1)*	a. A network of agencies, facilities, and providers involved with health care in a specified geographic area
_____ 2. healthcare system *(3)*	b. A disease or sickness that affects the body and/or mind
_____ 3. holistic health care *(3)*	c. To be without illness or in the absence of disease
_____ 4. health promotion *(2)*	d. Strategies that focus on prevention of injuries
_____ 5. illness *(1)*	e. Preventable differences in the effects of disease, injury, violence, that are experienced by socially disadvantaged populations
_____ 6. injury prevention *(2)*	f. The state of being in good physical and mental health
_____ 7. wellness *(3)*	g. A system of comprehensive or total patient care that considers the physical, emotional, social, economic, and spiritual needs of a person
_____ 8. health disparity *(1)*	h. Strategies that aim to keep a person healthy from the beginning

SHORT ANSWER

Directions: Using your own words, answer each question in the space provided.

9. Describe the focus of the *Healthy People* goals and objectives. *(1)*

_____

_____

_____

10. Define *health disparity* and provide examples. Describe potential causes of health disparities and potential ways to address health disparities. *(1)*

_____

_____

_____

11. Identify unforeseen consequences of the Affordable Care Act as it relates to the nursing shortage. *(2)*

_____

_____

_____

MULTIPLE CHOICE

Directions: Select the best answer(s) for each of the following questions.

12. Which are examples of *Healthy People* goals and objectives? *(1)*
    1. Increase vaccinations
    2. Provide birth control access
    3. Decrease unemployment
    4. Treatment of sleep disorders
    5. Treatment of eating disorders

13. A difference in the health status of groups of people because of their race or ethnicity, sexual identity, age, or socioeconomic status is called: *(1)*
    1. malpractice.
    2. a health disparity.
    3. discrimination.
    4. health bias.

14. Exercising at least 30 minutes a day to prevent being significantly overweight is an example of: *(2)*
    1. wellness.
    2. health disparity prevention.
    3. injury prevention.
    4. a health promotion strategy.

15. Wearing seatbelts is an example of: *(2)*
    1. wellness.
    2. health disparity prevention.
    3. injury prevention.
    4. a health promotion strategy.

16. The Affordable Care Act: *(2)*
    1. provides unlimited medical coverage.
    2. eliminates copays and coinsurance.
    3. prohibits denial of coverage based on preexisting conditions.
    4. requires employers to provide coverage for all employees.

17. Utilizing Maslow's hierarchy of needs, the patient care technician gives priority to which problem? *(3)*
    1. Loneliness due to being away from family during hospitalization
    2. Inability to eat because of difficulty chewing and swallowing
    3. Anxiety due to recent diagnosis of cancer with poor prognosis
    4. Safety related to difficulty with balance during position change

CRITICAL THINKING ACTIVITY

18. A patient is admitted to the medical-surgical unit for exacerbation of a chronic respiratory disease. While in the hospital, the patient requires medication, oxygen therapy, and diagnostic testing. In addition, the patient care technician notes that the patient smokes. He is overweight and making very poor food choices for between-meal snacks. He is unsteady when he ambulates and requires some assistance for activities that require bending and lifting, such as tying his shoelaces or picking up his suitcase. The patient care technician finds out that the patient lives by himself in a second-story apartment and his primary source of income is from a small pension.
    a. Identify all of the participants in the health care delivery system who will be involved in this patient's care and briefly describe their roles and responsibilities. *(4–5)*

    _____

    _____

    _____

    _____

    _____

b. What concepts of health promotion and illness prevention could assist this patient? *(3–4)*

_____

_____

_____

_____

_____

This page intentionally left blank

2 The Role of the Patient Care Technician

FILL IN THE BLANK SENTENCES

Directions: Complete each sentence by filling in the blank with the correct word or phrase.

1. Sandra should consider both the _____ and the _____ as she considers the various positions offered to her on graduation from her patient care technician training. (13, Figure 2-1)

2. Robert is anxious to learn _____, because he would like to draw blood and possibly work in a local hospital laboratory. (11)

3. It is important for graduates of patient care technician programs to gain _____ as soon as possible after graduation and maintain it throughout their patient care technician career. (11)

4. _____ may be required to maintain the patient care technician's certification. (13)

SHORT ANSWER

Directions: Using your own words, answer each question in the space provided.

5. Describe some of the benefits offered by employers in the medical field. (14)

_____

_____

_____

_____

_____

6. Name the two major areas of patient care technician practice. (10)

a. _____

b. _____

7. List five administrative duties a patient care technician might perform. (10)

a. _____

b. _____

c. _____

d. _____

e. _____

8. List five clinical duties a patient care technician might perform. (10)

a. _____

b. _____

c. _____

d. _____

e. _____

5

9. Explain why continuing education is critical to the success of the patient care technician. (13)

_____

_____

_____

_____

_____

10. Explain in your own words the history of the patient care technician. (11)

_____

_____

_____

_____

_____

_____

MULTIPLE CHOICE

Directions: Select the best answer(s) for each of the following questions.

11. Amber is occasionally assigned to work in different departments of the hospital where she has new and different tasks. This is an example of: (13)
    1. benefits.
    2. simulation.
    3. versatility.
    4. cross-training.

12. During orientation, the human resources manager highlights a new patient care technician's benefits package. Which would be considered job benefits? (*Select all that apply.*) (14)
    1. Paid time off
    2. Employer-provided cell phone
    3. Health care insurance
    4. Free continuing education units
    5. Travel opportunities

13. An area with growing utilization of patient care technicians is: (11)
    1. ultrasound.
    2. radiology.
    3. phlebotomy.
    4. hemodialysis.

14. The CNA is permitted to complete which of the following tasks? (*Select all that apply.*) (11, Table 2-1)
    1. Vital signs
    2. Hourly rounding
    3. Electrocardiogram (ECG)
    4. Urine diagnostic screenings
    5. Phlebotomy (fingersticks, venipuncture)

15. Good grooming for the patient care technician includes: (*Select all that apply.*) (14–15)
    1. styled fingernails.
    2. personal cleanliness.
    3. polished dress shoes.
    4. professionally applied makeup.
    5. moderate use of perfume and aftershave.

6

3 Professionalism and Work Ethics

FILL IN THE BLANK SENTENCES

Directions: Fill in the blanks with the correct vocabulary terms from this chapter.

1. Anna has worked as a patient care technician for almost 30 years, and her professionalism and compassion are above _____. (18)

2. _____ is one of the most important attributes that patient care technicians should display as they go about their duties. (18)

3. James has learned that he must use _____ when dealing with the patients in the clinic, being careful not to reveal any confidential information to an unauthorized third party. (20)

4. Roberta _____ the notes from the last staff meeting to all employees. (20)

5. Jessica holds drawings for small gifts at her staff meetings, which helps to raise employee _____. (20)

6. Gene evokes a professional _____ when talking with patients that encourages them to place their trust in him. (18)

7. Patient care technicians must take the _____ to look for opportunities to be of help when they are performing both externship and job duties. (18)

8. _____ is a cause for immediate dismissal from employment. (21)

9. The phrase "office politics" often has a negative _____. (21)

SHORT ANSWER

Directions: Using your own words, answer each question in the space provided.

10. Define *teamwork* in your own words. (21)

_____

_____

_____

_____

11. Karen has developed a friendship with Angela, who has a wonderful personality but does not always do her share in the family practice clinic where they work together. Dr. Rabinowitz tells Karen that Angela is going to be terminated on Friday, and she asks Karen to take over some of Angela's duties until a replacement is found. How can Karen demonstrate loyalty to her employer in this situation? How can she demonstrate loyalty to her friend Angela? (18)

_____

_____

_____

_____

12. Martin Smith is a patient who always disrupts the clinic. He constantly complains about everything from the moment he enters until the moment he leaves. Pamela is at the desk when he arrives to check out and pay his bill. When she tells him that he has a previous balance from a claim that his insurance did not pay, he argues that Pamela filed the claim incorrectly. Pamela is not in charge of filing insurance claims and did not handle any part of the claim in question. How can she be courteous to this patient? (17)

_____

_____

_____

13. Ming and her fiancé ended their relationship last week. How can she deal with personal stressors while she is in the workplace? (20)

_____

_____

_____

_____

14. A patient needs to be scheduled for an outpatient endoscopic examination. When Victor gives the instruction sheet to the patient, he suspects from the patient's reaction that she is unable to read. How can Victor professionally handle this situation without causing embarrassment to the patient? (23)

_____

_____

_____

_____

15. List five obstructions to professionalism. Which of the five obstructions to professionalism will be most difficult for you to overcome? Explain why. (20–21)

_____

_____

_____

16. Explain the difference between drug abuse and drug addiction. (23)

_____

_____

_____

_____

MULTIPLE CHOICE

Directions: Select the best answer(s) for each of the following questions.

17. Karen works in the office laboratory. She is often asked questions about insurance and billing. Despite this not being her usual task or responsibility, Karen gathered relevant insurance and billing handouts for patients and has taken note of the responses for the most common inquiries so she can assist patients as much as possible. This is an example of: (18–19)
    1. positive attitude.
    2. flexibility.
    3. prioritizing.
    4. credibility.

18. *Working smart* can be described as: (21)
    1. using your time efficiently and concentrating on the most important duties first.
    2. the inclination to put the most favorable construction on actions and anticipating the best outcome possible.
    3. causing or facilitating the start of something or to cause something to happen.
    4. having the ability to adapt to a wide variety of situations.

19. Initiative can be described as: (18)
    1. the ability to adapt to a wide variety of situations.
    2. the inclination to put the most favorable construction on actions and events or to anticipate the best possible outcome.
    3. having the energy or aptitude to cause or facilitate the start of something or to cause something to happen.
    4. an individual's social façade or front that reflects the role in life the individual is playing.

20. Optimism can be described as: (19)
    1. having adequate or requisite capabilities.
    2. the quality or power of inspiring belief.
    3. anticipating the best possible outcome.
    4. an expression of rebuke or disapproval.

21. A patient's family member inquires about the patient's medical condition. The patient care technician should confirm which of the following before providing the requested information? (19)
    1. A signed release applicable to third parties is on file.
    2. No one can overhear the conversation.
    3. The nurse approves providing the information to the relative.
    4. The person is a relative.

9

This page intentionally left blank

4 Communicating with the Healthcare Team

FILL IN THE BLANK SENTENCES

Directions: Complete each sentence by filling in the blank with the correct word or phrase.

1. Accurate _____ is one of the best defenses in the event of legal claims associated with patient care. (30)

2. Auditors are appointed to examine patient charts and health records to assess _____. (30)

3. The denotative meaning is the _____ definition of a particular word. (26)

4. _____ is the process of recording the interventions carried out to meet the patient's needs. (30)

5. _____ is a classification system of technical or scientific names and terminology. (31)

6. SBAR stands for _____. (32)

SHORT ANSWER

Directions: Using your own words, answer each question in the space provided.

7. Take a moment to think about your natural communication style. How do you respond in stressful situations? How do you react to those who are combative or abrasive? How can your communication style positively and negatively impact your interactions with colleagues and patients? (28–29)

_____

_____

_____

_____

8. The five basic purposes of written patient records are: (30)_____

_____

_____

_____

9. Describe narrative charting. (33)_____

_____

_____

_____

MULTIPLE CHOICE

Directions: Select the best answer(s) for each of the following questions.

10. Tina is caring for a patient who just had a cholecystectomy (gallbladder removal surgery). The patient refuses to have her dressings changed, saying that she is afraid that her wound will be "aggravated" if they "start messing around with it." Tina makes direct eye contact and explains why it's important to change the patient's dressings. She explains each step in the dressing change and also addresses the patient's pain concerns. Which communication style best describes Tina's response in this situation? (28, Box 4-1)
    1. Nonverbal communication
    2. One-way communication
    3. Aggressive communication
    4. Assertive communication

11. The patient care technician is giving report during shift change. A visitor passing by is an unintended receiver. What is the best method to prevent this type of occurrence? (26)
    1. Ask visitors to leave the unit during shift change.
    2. Give report in a private room with the door closed.
    3. Eliminate negative connotations during report.
    4. Make written notes that are passed only to staff members.

12. Which describes a situation in which someone receives a message differently from how the sender meant it to be received? (26)
    1. Denotative meaning
    2. Connotative meaning
    3. Aggressive communication
    4. Assertive communication

13. Nonverbal communication includes: (*Select all that apply.*) (27)
    1. jargon.
    2. clothing.
    3. posture.
    4. gestures.
    5. tone of voice.

14. When communicating with a patient of an unfamiliar culture, the patient care technician knows that: (*Select all that apply.*) (27)
    1. gestures can have different meanings.
    2. characteristics of people's voices can vary.
    3. smiling and handshakes are universal greetings.
    4. tone of voice should be soft and deferential.
    5. eye contact has different meaning among cultures.

15. The student patient care technician sees that it is time to give medication to a patient, but the patient is currently in X-ray. The student is aware that there is a 30-minute time window to administer the medication, otherwise it will be considered late. What should the student do? (32, Box 4-2)
    1. Document that the medication was given at the correct time and then give it as soon as the patient returns from X-ray.
    2. Call the pharmacy and inquire if a delay in administering the medication or holding it until the next dose is harmful to the patient.
    3. Document that the patient is in X-ray, advise the nurse, and administer the medication when the patient returns to the unit.
    4. Hold the medication and fill out an incident report that explains the circumstances and details of why the medication was not administered.

16. Once home, Aaron, the patient care technician, remembers that he forgot to document some items in his patient's chart. He calls the health center and speaks with Sara, the patient care technician now caring for the patient and informs Sara of the items he neglected to document. After their phone call, Sara updates the patient's chart with the information Aaron provided with no additional explanations. Which was an inappropriate action? (32, Box 4-2)
    1. Charting after care was provided, not before
    2. Failing to note that this was a late entry
    3. Charting for a colleague
    4. Breaching patient confidentiality

17. Carrie is mentoring Samantha, a new patient care technician. Which is appropriate advice for safe computer documentation? (41, Box 4-3)
    1. Provide all passwords to your supervisor.
    2. Contact IT as soon as possible if files are accidentally deleted.
    3. Shred printouts of patient records.
    4. Log out of the computer whenever anyone is around.

18. A patient is grimacing while trying to reposition himself in bed. He tells the patient care technician that he is feeling great and is ready to get up and go home. Which response best indicates that the patient care technician recognizes that the patient's communication is incongruent? (28)
    1. "Going home is the goal, but let me help you get up and you can walk around for a while."
    2. "Let me help you sit up and then you can get dressed and pack up your belongings."
    3. "Would you like a dose of pain medication before you go home?"
    4. "That sounds great! I'll call your health care provider and inform her that you are ready to go home."

19. An auditor is randomly reviewing the patient charts and the nurse manager has agreed that the auditor can ask questions and give feedback as necessary. Which documentation is the auditor mostly likely to query? (30)
    1. Ambulated independently with steady gait to bathroom.
    2. Instructed on method of clean midstream urine collection.
    3. Discharged to home accompanied by spouse.
    4. Placed side rails up ×3 with call bell in place.

20. In using the hospital's computer information system, where would the patient care technician most likely find documentation about the patient's response to the last dose of pain medication? (33)
    1. Individualized care plan
    2. Medication administration record (MAR)
    3. Automated Kardex form
    4. Narrative notes

21. The patient care technician is working on a medical-surgical unit in a large hospital and observes an unfamiliar person looking at a patient's chart. What should the patient care technician do? (38–39)
    1. Call hospital security and report the person's behavior and description.
    2. Ask for identification and determine if the person can look at the chart.
    3. Allow the person to continue unless there is suspicious behavior.
    4. Request that the chart be returned and contact the nurse.

22. The patient care technician is being advised by an auditor about possible inadequate or inappropriate documentation that could be involved in a malpractice suit. What type(s) of documentation is/are likely to cause problems in malpractice cases? (*Select all that apply.*) (32, Box 4-2)
    1. Failed to document latex allergy.
    2. Documented patient's complaint about care by using patient's remarks in quotes.
    3. Charted medication that patient claims he did not receive.
    4. Documented amount of IV fluid, but no assessment of IV site.
    5. Clustered information obtained from physical assessment.
    6. Recorded verbal order using brand-name medication.

23. Which action/behavior would be considered a potential HIPAA violation on the part of the patient care technician? (38)
    1. Faxes a patient's medical records to a consulting specialist
    2. Leaves the computer monitor display open for easy access
    3. Discusses a patient problem during handover with oncoming staff
    4. Documents contents of an SBARR report for the risk manager

24. A patient approaches the patient care technician and demands to have his chart because he has decided to leave the hospital and seek care from a different facility. What is the best response? (38)
    1. "Sir, all of the patient records are the property of the hospital."
    2. "Sir, let me contact your health care provider so you can talk to him before leaving."
    3. "Sir, please wait and I will call the nurse right now."
    4. "Sir, please return to your room and I will make a copy of the chart."

5 Understanding the Patient as a Person

FILL IN THE BLANK SENTENCES

Directions: Complete each sentence by filling in the blank with the correct word or phrase.

1. _____ refers to the degree to which people can understand basic health information in order to make their own decisions about treatment options. (48)

2. _____ means that the patient care technician is aware of his or her own cultural beliefs and practices and how they relate to those of others, which may be different. (45)

3. A(n) _____ is a generalized expectation about forms of behavior, an individual, or a group. (45)

4. In the United States, the largest increase has occurred in the _____ population, which rose from 16.3% to 18.7% between 2010 and 2020. (Table 5.1)

5. Western cultures generally use the _____ which may have limitations when used to develop a plan of care for culturally diverse patients with different health beliefs. (54)

MULTIPLE CHOICE

Directions: Select the best answer(s) for each of the following questions.

6. When communicating with a patient who has limited understanding of English, the patient care technician should: (47)
   1. speak loudly to emphasize key information.
   2. keep questions brief and simple.
   3. use sign language and get an interpreter.
   4. provide detailed directions.

7. What cultural difference(s) does the patient care technician need to be aware of when caring for an older adult? (*Select all that apply.*) (45)
   1. They are more tolerant of other cultures.
   2. They may say hurtful things if cognitive impairment is present.
   3. They are more likely to be rigid in their practices.
   4. They are less likely to use home remedies.
   5. They rely more on traditional religious practices.
   6. They are less likely to be well-educated.

8. The health care provider informs the patient that there is a risk of blood loss during the planned surgical procedure, but the patient is a Jehovah's Witness, so she refuses to sign the consent form. Which action does the patient care technician expect the nurse to take in the best interest of the patient? (Box 5.5)
   1. Support the patient's decision to refuse the procedure.
   2. Discuss realistic alternatives to blood transfusion with the health care provider.
   3. Document the patient's decision in the medical record.
   4. Contact the risk manager for advice about convincing the patient.

9. A patient who is a Muslim American dies during the night. What action should the patient care technician perform in order to respect the patient's religious beliefs? (Box 5.5)
   1. Contact the family before giving any postmortem care.
   2. Stay with the deceased until a family member arrives.
   3. Wait at least 30 minutes before giving postmortem care.
   4. Contact the organ transplant team because donation is likely.

10. The patient care technician is from a small town in the southern United States and is starting a new job in a large urban area with a diverse population. What strategy(ies) can the patient care technician use to develop cultural competence? (*Select all that apply.*) (45)
    1. Perform a self-assessment of beliefs and practices.
    2. Adapt personal beliefs to match those of individual patients.
    3. Keep an open mind about cultural differences.
    4. Treat everyone as equal and act the same toward all patients.
    5. Ignore the differences and focus on exhibiting kindness and care.
    6. Understand his or her own values, preferences, and cultural heritage.

11. The patient care technician is trying to explain the importance of taking blood pressure medication every day to an older patient who is on a fixed income. Which question from the patient suggests that his perception of time tends to be present-oriented? (49)
   1. "Can I save the medication on the days when I feel okay?"
   2. "What should I do if I am running out of medication and have no money?"
   3. "My wife takes blood pressure medication too. Can I share her pills?"
   4. "Would you take this medication if you were in my position?"

12. The patient care technician is discussing the parents' beliefs and use of folk medicine, which they would like to use in the treatment of their child's respiratory infection. Which health care practice is the cause of greatest concern? (54)
   1. Placing a religious medal on the bedside table
   2. Having a folk healer come to heal with touch and faith
   3. Giving the child an herbal tea that gives strength and health
   4. Bathing at night instead of in the morning

13. On visiting the patient at home with the nurse, they find that the patient is not following the dietary instructions. The wife states that she does the grocery shopping and cooks under the belief that her husband needs "nutritious home-cooked meals from his native country." What does the patient care technician expect the nurse to do first? (54)
   1. Change the dietary plan to meet the patient's and family's cultural preferences.
   2. Consult a nutritionist for ways to adapt the wife's cooking to the dietary plan.
   3. Revise the patient's nutritional goal to incorporate the cultural dietary patterns.
   4. Ask the wife to describe a typical 24-hour day of meal preparation and snacks.

CRITICAL THINKING ACTIVITY

14. The patient care technician is caring for an older patient who has recently emigrated from another country. The patient's family is at the bedside and the patient care technician overhears them speaking in English and Spanish. The patient care technician's first language is English and she understands and speaks a little Spanish.
   a. Identify strategies that may be used to communicate with a non–English-speaking patient. (Box 5.2)

   _____
   _____

   b. Discuss the advantages and disadvantages of using a family member to translate and communicate with the patient. (47)

   _____
   _____
   _____
   _____
   _____
   _____
   _____

   c. How should the nurse ask the patient about the following? (47; Box 5.2)

   i. Language: _____

   ii. Health: _____

   iii. Family structure: _____

   iv. Dietary practices: _____

   v. Use of folk medicine: _____

6 Patient Rights, Ethics, and Laws

MATCHING

Directions: Match the terms on the left to the correct definition on the right.

Terms	Definitions
1. abandonment of care (Box 6.3)	a. Injury that gives basis for a legal action against the person who caused the damage
2. accountability (62)	b. Failure to perform the duty in a reasonable, prudent manner
3. breach of duty (60)	c. Professional negligence
4. proximate cause (60)	d. Being responsible for one's own actions
5. competency (Box 6.3)	e. Wrongful termination of providing patient care
6. harm (Box 6.3)	f. Legal presumption that a person can make decisions for him- or herself unless proven otherwise
7. malpractice (Box 6.3)	g. Defines acts whose performance is required, permitted, or prohibited
8. negligence (Box 6.3)	h. Occurrence of harm depended directly on the occurrence of the breach
9. standards of care (62)	i. Legal responsibility
10. liability (62)	j. Absence of due care

TRUE OR FALSE

Directions: Write T for true or F for false in the blanks provided.

11. The purpose of civil law is to *make the aggrieved person whole again*, to restore the person to where he or she was. (Box 6.1)

12. The purpose of criminal law is to *punish* for the crime and deter and *prevent* further crimes. (Box 6.1)

13. The duty to care for the patient exists when the nurse accepts a position at a facility. (60)

14. The nurse who uses unnecessary restraints on a patient may be charged with assault. (Box 6.3)

15. When providing first aid in an emergency situation outside a medical facility, it is important for the nurse to have knowledge of the Good Samaritan Act. (67)

MULTIPLE CHOICE

Directions: Select the best answer(s) for each of the following questions.

16. The patient care technician student needs to obtain patient information to prepare for the clinical experience and decides to stop and say hello to the patient. While they are talking, the patient suddenly stops breathing and becomes unresponsive. What should the student do first? (60)
    1. Call the nursing instructor and write an incident report.
    2. Call the primary nurse and apply oxygen.
    3. Call the Rapid Response Team and get the crash cart.
    4. Call for help and initiate CPR.

17. In which case is the patient care technician most likely to be charged with malpractice? (60)
    1. The patient care technician explains the restraint policy to the family and later the elderly patient climbs over the side rail and sustains a hip fracture.
    2. The patient becomes very angry when the patient care technician refuses to give an additional dose of pain medication before the ordered time.
    3. The family wants the health care provider called at 3:00 AM because "something is wrong." The patient care technician waits until 7:00 AM, but the patient is unharmed.
    4. The patient is very demanding and unpleasant, so the patient care technician ignores the call bell; the patient sustains tissue injury at the IV site.

18. The patient asked the patient care technician to apply a heating pad to her back, despite the fact that the nurse had instructed both patient and technician to avoid using the device. The patient sustained a burn and decided to sue the patient care technician and the nurse. Which document(s) is/are likely to be used in this case? (*Select all that apply.*) (Box 6.5)
    1. Policies and procedures
    2. Standards of care
    3. Equipment maintenance records
    4. Patient's medical records
    5. Patient care technician's personal health records
    6. Personnel files for the patient care technician and nurse

19. The patient care technician recognizes that in today's health care climate, there is an increased likelihood to be involved in litigation. What action could the patient care technician take to improve the overall situation in the work setting? (62)
    1. Agree to take a limited number of high-acuity patients.
    2. Work on a committee to improve discharge teaching.
    3. Work at a facility that covers patient care technicians with malpractice insurance.
    4. Ensure that others are accountable for their own actions.

20. A new patient care technician is assigned to do a task that was reviewed and demonstrated in orientation and practiced on a mannequin. The patient care technician tells the nurse that she does not know how to do the task. What would the patient care technician expect the nurse to do first? (Delegation and Documentation Box 6.1)
    1. Ask the patient care technician to recite the steps of the task and assess readiness to perform.
    2. Go with the patient care technician and perform the task while she observes.
    3. Instruct the patient care technician to try to perform the task to the best of her ability.
    4. Pull the patient care technician's orientation file and see if competency was established.

21. A patient care technician student must write a clinical report about the care that was given to a patient in the hospital. What should the student do to prevent a HIPAA violation? (Select all that apply.) (64)
    1. Do not use the patient's name in any section of the paper.
    2. If laboratory data are used, make sure no identification numbers are included.
    3. Avoid including the health care provider's name in the report.
    4. Do not refer to the room number or the specific unit.
    5. Do not include the patient's vital signs.
    6. Avoid using specific details of the patient's medical condition.

22. Which unaccompanied minor requires parental consent prior to treatment? (64)
    1. A 17-year-old who wants a prescription for insulin
    2. An 18-year-old who needs sutures for a laceration to the hand
    3. A 14-year-old who was sexually assaulted by a family member
    4. A 16-year-old who is independent and self-supporting and wants birth control

23. The patient care technician is working on the medical-surgical unit and answers the telephone. The caller wants to know, "How is Mr. Smith doing?" What is the most important factor that affects the response? (66)
    1. The identity of the caller
    2. The stability of Mr. Smith's condition
    3. The hospital's policy for releasing information
    4. The patient care technician's knowledge of HIPAA

24. A mother brings her 8-year-old son to the clinic for a broken arm. There are no other apparent injuries and the child and mother appear to have a supportive relationship; however, review of the chart indicates that this child has frequently been treated for other fractures and injuries. What should the patient care technician do first? (66)
    1. Ask the social worker to consult for possible child abuse.
    2. Call child protective services and make a report.
    3. Point out the history of injuries to the health care provider.
    4. Take the child aside and assess his true feelings.

25. The patient care technician is working in the emergency department. There is a gunshot sound from the waiting room, followed by sounds of yelling and screaming. What should the technician do first? (67)
    1. Grab the crash cart and run to the waiting room.
    2. Reassure all of the patients in the immediate area.
    3. Call 911 and the hospital's security personnel.
    4. Lock the entrance to patient care areas.

26. Which action by the patient care technician is the best step to avoid a lawsuit? (67)
    1. Provide compassionate, competent care.
    2. Know the legal definition of terms, such as *negligence*.
    3. Obtain professional malpractice insurance.
    4. Validate patient care actions with a supervisor.

27. The patient care technician performs a dressing change on a surgical wound. The procedure is routine and there are no signs of infection or excessive drainage. What should the patient care technician do about documentation? (67)
    1. If using charting by exception, "dressing changed" is adequate.
    2. Document appearance of wound site and type of dressing used.
    3. There is no need to document, because there are no problems with the wound.
    4. Read the previous entry about the wound and document "unchanged as above."

28. An elderly patient begins to cry during the review of the advance directive information and refuses to sign. What should the patient care technician do first? (67)
    1. Encourage the patient to express his feelings about the advance directives.
    2. Reassure the patient that his wishes will be respected above all else.
    3. Alert the family to support the patient in the decision.
    4. Document in the patient's record that the information was given and declined.

29. A patient is in very critical condition and unable to make decisions about ongoing treatment. There is conflict among family members on what should be done. Which source, if followed, is the most likely to protect the health care team from liability? (68)
    1. Agency's policy and procedure manual
    2. Patient's living will
    3. Patient Self-Determination Act
    4. Accreditation criteria of the Joint Commission

30. A mother and her pregnant 13-year-old daughter are arguing; the mother wants her to keep the baby and the girl wants to have an abortion. The patient care technician feels very angry toward the mother and very protective toward the girl. What should the technician do first? (68-69)
    1. Take the girl aside and assess her feelings and wishes regarding the pregnancy.
    2. Ask another nurse to assess the mother's rationale for opposing her daughter.
    3. Seek advice from a supervisor about who can legally make decisions about the pregnancy.
    4. Reflect on own feelings and ability to be supportive and caring toward this family.

CRITICAL THINKING ACTIVITY

31. A new patient care technician has just started his first job after graduating. The patient care technician sees a health care provider's order to "get surgical consent form," but he is unsure what the order means, so he calls the health care provider for clarification. The provider is a little terse on the phone and says, "just get the consent form signed." The patient care technician consults the nurse who says, "Oh, the doctors here are too lazy to get their own consent forms signed, so we always do it for them." (64)
    a. Discuss the nurse's responsibilities when obtaining an informed consent from a patient before a procedure.

    _____

    _____

    _____

    _____

    b. The patient care technician is new to the city and this is his first job, so he has limited experience, but he clearly remembers what was taught in school about informed consent. What should he do?

    _____

    _____

    _____

    _____

This page intentionally left blank

7 Body Structure and Function/ Growth and Development

MATCHING

Directions: Match the terms on the left to the correct definition or characteristics on the right.

Terms	Definition or Characteristics
_____ 1. adoptive family (Box 7-2)	a. Grandparents, grandchildren, aunts, and uncles living in the same household
_____ 2. nuclear family (Box 7-2)	b. Family with adopted children
_____ 3. extended family (Box 7-2)	c. Children may have loyalties to one parent
_____ 4. single-parent family (Box 7-2)	d. Same-sex couple
_____ 5. blended family (Box 7-2)	e. Parents and their biologic offspring
_____ 6. cohabitation (Box 7-2)	f. Unmarried couple living together and sharing responsibilities
_____ 7. homosexual family (Box 7-2)	g. Result of death, divorce, separation, or abandonment
_____ 8. grandfamilies (Box 7-2)	h. Children may "age out" of system
_____ 9. foster family (Box 7-2)	i. Related to increase of substance abuse, mental illness, military deployment, incarceration, and parental death

TRUE OR FALSE

Directions: Write T for true or F for false in the blanks provided.

_____ 10. It is estimated that a possible 5–25% of unfavorable outcomes in all pregnancies are attributable to smoking. (86)

_____ 11. Infants will speak spontaneously. (89)

_____ 12. The adolescent often requires fewer hours of sleep because of hormonal surge. (103)

_____ 13. Many older adults choose to work after age 65 years. (110)

_____ 14. The fastest-growing segment of the U.S. population is the group aged 65 years and older. (107)

SHORT ANSWER

Directions: Using your own words, answer each question in the space provided.

15. Identify factors that have contributed to the changes that families of today have undergone and are still undergoing. (Box 7-1)

_____

_____

16. Discuss the qualities of functional families. (Box 7-3)_____

_____

_____

17. Three common causes of family stress are: (88)_____

_____

_____

TABLE ACTIVITY

18. Directions: Insert the expected values of vital signs for different age groups. (91, 94, 97, 98, 101)

Age Group	Temperature	Pulse	Respirations (at Rest)	Blood Pressure
Infants at 12 months				
Toddler 1–3 years				
Preschool 3–5 years				
School age 6–12 years				
Adolescent 12–19 years				

MULTIPLE CHOICE

Directions: Select the best answer(s) for each of the following questions.

19. Which action(s) contribute(s) to accomplishing the *Healthy People 2020* Health Indicators? (*Select all that apply.* (Table 7-7)
    1. Administers medication on time using the 6 rights
    2. Reinforces the need for preventive dental care
    3. Encourages patients to routinely exercise
    4. Assists patients to locate smoking cessation literature
    5. Shows respect and courtesy to elderly patients
    6. Teaches patients how to limit fats and sugar in the diet

20. Most of the weight gain in the first months of life is in the form of fat. What is the best physiologic explanation for this gain of fat? (37)
    1. Fat provides insulation and a source of nourishment if teething or other problems decrease food intake for a few days.
    2. In cephalocaudal growth, fat must be deposited in areas of the trunk and abdomen before growth in extremities can occur.
    3. Breast milk or prepared formulas are high in nutrients that are more readily converted to fat than to muscle or bone tissue.
    4. Muscle and bone require more protein and calcium, so development of these tissues is concurrent with intake of solid foods.

21. The mother of a 5-month-old infant reports the child is irritable; gums are red and edematous, and he demonstrates excessive drooling. What does the patient care technician expect the nurse to recommend? (91)
    1. Advise the mother to contact the health care provider for treatment of infection.
    2. Suggest the mother wipe and massage the gums and offer sips of clear water.
    3. Teach the mother to brush the gums with a soft brush and fluoride toothpaste.
    4. Advise the mother to give an infant dose of acetaminophen for discomfort.

22. The patient care technician would advise the parents to contact the health care provider if their 1-year-old infant: (93)
    1. seems restless and makes little noises during short naplike periods.
    2. cries persistently during usual sleep periods and is inconsolable.
    3. sleeps 12 hours a night and takes one nap during the day.
    4. frequently kicks and stretches when in the supine position.

23. The working mother has an 8-month-old child who has to go to daycare while she works. How can the patient care technician best help the mother prepare for the first day of daycare? (91)
    1. Explain the likelihood of separation anxiety as a normal behavior.
    2. Emphasize that the child is likely to sleep most of the day, so he won't miss her.
    3. Describe the benefits of parallel play for cognitive development.
    4. Validate the mother's feelings of guilt and reassure that daycare is beneficial.

24. The patient care technician is watching a group of mothers interact with their young children. Which behavior by a mother would most suggest that additional assessment for potential child abuse might be required? (89 and 95)
    1. Retrieves toddler whenever he tries to run or jump or perform active movements
    2. Allows toddler to climb on a table space that is meant for snacks and drinks
    3. Berates and shames her toddler for refusing to share toys with other children
    4. Talks to other mothers and allows the toddler to fuss without comforting him

25. The patient care technician is interviewing the parents of a toddler who must be admitted for 23-hour observation for a febrile illness. What would be the most important question to ask about the child's bedtime? (96)
   1. "Would you prefer that he gets milk or juice in a night bottle?"
   2. "What do you usually do when you put him to bed?"
   3. "How many hours does he usually sleep?"
   4. "What would you like me to tell him about sleeping away from home?"

26. The mother is ordering lunch for her toddler. The patient care technician would intervene if the mother selected which food for the toddler? (95–96)
   1. Milk
   2. Peanut butter sandwich
   3. Carrot sticks
   4. Small banana

27. The parents report that their 3-year-old child has not started talking, but he seems happy and active and very interactive with the world in nonverbal ways. What does the patient care technician expect the nurse to advise the parents to do? (97)
   1. Advise the parents to read to the child and ask him to name familiar objects.
   2. Suggest expanding opportunities for parallel play, such as at daycare or play groups.
   3. Reassure parents that children grow and develop at their own individual pace.
   4. Suggest consultation with the health care provider for possible hearing or speech problems.

28. The health care provider tells the nurse that he has to privately talk to the mother and asks if the patient care technician would please watch the 4-year-old child. What would be the best way for the patient care technician to interact with the child? (97)
   1. Take the child to the cafeteria and buy him a snack.
   2. Give him some crayons and paper and ask him to draw a picture.
   3. Ask him to "help" by sorting a bag of rubber bands by size and color.
   4. Explain why he has to wait and give him a book to read.

29. The patient care technician must give the school-age child an immunization. Based on the patient care technician's awareness that the child is in the concrete operational stage, what would the patient care technician do prior to giving the child the injection? (99)
   1. Ask a helper to hold the child to prevent movement.
   2. Suggest that the child pretend that she is getting a fairy's kiss.
   3. Tell the child that it hurts a bit, but prevents sickness.
   4. Make extra efforts to protect modesty and privacy.

30. Which routine check-up(s) or screening(s) is/are recommended for school-age children? (*Select all that apply.*) (98)
   1. Vision testing
   2. Dental examination every 6 months
   3. Hearing testing
   4. Scoliosis screening
   5. Cancer screening
   6. HIV testing

31. The patient care technician must perform a dressing change on a 7-year-old child. The patient care technician explains that the procedure will not be painful, but the child appears apprehensive. What is the best approach for the patient care technician to use? (99)
   1. Demonstrate the procedure on a doll and answer questions.
   2. Ask the child to hold the tape strips and praise her.
   3. Premedicate with a mild anxiolytic medication and explain.
   4. Coach the parent through the procedure and stand back.

32. A parent expresses concern because her 11-year-old healthy, active son seems very short. She reports that all men on both sides of the family are tall. What is the best information that the patient care technician can give to the mother about growth and development? (*Select all that apply.* (98)
   1. During the school-age period, the growth pattern is usually gradual and subtle.
   2. A second period of rapid growth is expected during adolescence.
   3. From ages 6 to 12, height increases by about 2 inches.
   4. He is probably lacking essential nutrients that contribute to height and weight.
   5. Distant genetic factors are likely to predispose him to a shorter height.

Chapter **7** **Body Structure and Function/Growth and Development**

33. Developmental tasks of early adulthood include: (*Select all that apply.*) (Box 7-18)
    1. achieving financial and social independence.
    2. accepting self and others.
    3. maximizing personal worth and identity.
    4. making decisions regarding career, marriage, and children.
    5. developing own value system.

34. Which behavior demonstrates that a 55-year-old adult is meeting his developmental task of generativity? (105)
    1. Ruminates over fears and lifetime failures
    2. Reorganizes personal belongings and assets
    3. Gives advice to nephew about succeeding in life
    4. Reviews will for distribution of worldly goods

35. The patient care technician is assisting the nurse who is assessing the vision of an older adult patient. Which finding is not associated with the aging process? (Table 7–10)
    1. Presbyopia
    2. Visualization of half the field
    3. Decreased depth perception
    4. Slowed accommodation

36. The patient care technician is working in a long-term care facility. Which activity will help the residents meet the developmental task of ego integrity as described by Erikson? (110)
    1. Taking the residents out to lunch at a restaurant
    2. Reminiscing about past important events
    3. Assisting residents to maintain personal hygiene
    4. Leading the residents in an arts and crafts project

CRITICAL THINKING ACTIVITIES

37. A young mother expresses frustration because she is having trouble toilet training her 18-month-old child. She reports that the child shows no interest in learning to use the "potty chair." She tells you that she has tried to sit the child on the potty chair and instructed the child to "urinate." She says that child frequently has temper tantrums when she places him on the chair.
    a. What can you tell the mother about physiologic development related to toilet training? (95)

    _____

    _____

    _____

    b. Use Erikson's stages of psychosocial development to explain how the mother can respond to the child during toilet training. (95)

    _____

    _____

    _____

    c. What can you tell the mother about the child's temper tantrums? (95)

    _____

    _____

    _____

38. The patient care technician is working in an assisted-living facility. The majority of the residents are elderly and have some chronic health problems; however, many of the residents are active and only manifest changes associated with aging. Describe the physical changes that the technician might observe in each of the following systems as a result of the aging process. (Table 7–10)

a. Sensory: _____

_____

b. Integumentary: _____

_____

c. Cardiovascular: _____

_____

d. Respiratory: _____

_____

e. Gastrointestinal: _____

_____

f. Genitourinary: _____

_____

g. Musculoskeletal: _____

_____

h. Neurologic: _____

_____

39. What influence does the aging process in late adulthood have on the following? (1007)

a. Ability to cope: _____

_____

b. Intelligence and learning: _____

_____

c. Memory: _____

_____

8 Pain Management, Comfort, Rest, and Sleep

FILL IN THE BLANK SENTENCES

Directions: Complete each sentence by filling in the blank with the correct word or phrase.

1. Pain is an unpleasant sensation caused by _____ stimulation of the sensory nerve endings. (115)
2. Treating pain as a(n) _____ increases the likelihood that it will be properly treated. (116)
3. Acute pain is intense and of short duration, usually lasting less than _____ months. (115)
4. The combination of fatigue, sleep disturbance, and depression has the potential to markedly change a person's _____ of pain. (116)
5. Pain relief measures such as transcutaneous electric nerve stimulation (TENS), acupuncture, and placebos are believed to cause the release of _____. (117)

TRUE OR FALSE

Directions: Write T for true or F for false in the blanks provided.

_____ 6. A predictable relationship exists between identifiable tissue injury and the sensation of pain. (115)

_____ 7. Certain invasive techniques offer relief for many patients with pain. (118)

_____ 8. The patient care technician should inform the nurse of patient complaints of pain immediately. (117)

_____ 9. Bedrest does not necessarily mean a patient is resting. (121)

_____ 10. Older adults require less sleep than younger people, but they are more likely to take naps. (122)

MULTIPLE CHOICE

Directions: Select the best answer(s) for each of the following questions.

11. The patient had a surgical procedure this morning and is requesting pain medication. The nurse assesses the patient's vital signs and decides to withhold opioid medication based on the finding of: (119)
    1. pulse = 90/min.
    2. respirations = 10/min.
    3. blood pressure = 130/80 mm Hg.
    4. temperature = 99° F rectally.

12. An emergency department patient is complaining of shortness of breath and shoulder pain. Later, it is determined that the patient had a heart attack. The shoulder pain is referred to as: (115)
    1. acute pain.
    2. chronic pain.
    3. referred pain.
    4. fight-or-flight response.

13. Which is the most common side effect of opioids? (118)
    1. Suicide risk
    2. Constipation
    3. Depressed immune response
    4. Increased oxygen demand

14. What are the benefits of the intravenous route for pain medication administration? (*Select all that apply.*) (118)
    1. Convenient
    2. Flexible
    3. Treats pain rapidly rising in intensity
    4. Produces relatively steady blood levels

15. Which action demonstrates compliance with the Joint Commission (TJC) standards of pain management? (116)
    1. Documents that medication is given after the patient receives it.
    2. Incorporates knowledge of the patient's culture in pain management.
    3. Assesses the patient's pain and reassesses pain after interventions.
    4. Stays current with the latest information about pain therapies.

16. The patient care technician reports to the nurse that a postoperative patient is asking for pain medication. What is the most important question that the nurse will ask the patient care technician? (116)
    1. "Can you give the medication yourself?"
    2. "What did the patient tell you about his pain?"
    3. "Did you try any nonpharmacologic interventions?"
    4. "What do you know about the ordered medication?"

17. The patient agrees to try guided imagery as a noninvasive method of pain relief. Before beginning the therapy, which instruction is the nurse most likely to give? (117)
    1. "I'll use a combination of firm and light strokes during the therapy."
    2. "The skin will be stimulated with a mild electric current that reduces pain."
    3. "Tell me about a place and time where you felt relaxed and peaceful."
    4. "We have to use specialized equipment to identify your biologic responses."

18. What is the greatest advantage of using noninvasive pain management techniques as an adjunct to pain medication? (117)
    1. Inexpensive and easy to perform
    2. Based on the gate control theory
    3. Low risk and few side effects
    4. Gives patients some control over pain

19. The patient care technician is talking to a patient who wants to try transcutaneous electric nerve stimulation (TENS). The patient care technician would alert the health care provider if the patient reveals he has a: (117)
    1. cardiac pacemaker device.
    2. hearing aid.
    3. metallic hip joint.
    4. history of a broken back.

20. The nurse is talking to an older adult who reports feeling tired and not getting enough sleep. Which question related to the patient's medication is most relevant to designing interventions for the patient's problem? (122)
    1. "Which NSAID medication has the health care provider suggested?"
    2. "Has there been a recent increase in the dosage of your opioid medication?"
    3. "What time of the day do you usually take your diuretic medication?"
    4. "Are you taking your antiemetic medication before or after meals?"

21. The new patient care technician is looking at jobs to consider after graduation. Which shift is most likely to cause the technician to have sleep-wake cycle disruption? (122)
    1. Straight night shift
    2. Rotating day to night shift
    3. Weekends-only evening shift
    4. Monday to Friday day shift

CRITICAL THINKING ACTIVITIES

22. a. The patient has identified to the nurse that she is experiencing pain. What does the patient care technician expect the nurse to do to fully assess the patient's pain? (115)

    _____

    _____

    b. What problem(s) can occur if the patient's pain is not relieved? (117)

    _____

    _____

c. Identify interventions that may be implemented to reduce or eliminate the patient's pain. (117–119; Table 8-1)

_____

_____

_____

_____

_____

23. The patient is experiencing difficulty sleeping while in the hospital. She reports this is the first time she has been in the hospital and the sounds and smells seem very strange. In addition, she reports feeling mildly anxious because "so many people come in and out of the room at all hours of the day and night." She looks tired and seems mildly irritable.

a. Identify and briefly describe the usual phases and stages of the sleep cycle and describe what is happening to patient when NREM and REM sleep are interrupted. (120–122; Box 8-2)

_____

_____

_____

b. Identify interventions that may be implemented to promote sleep. (123) _____

_____

_____

_____

29

This page intentionally left blank

9 Asepsis and Infection Control

TRUE OR FALSE

Directions: Write T for true or F for false in the blanks provided.

_____ 1. Following isolation precautions is the most important method of reducing the spread of microorganisms. (129)

_____ 2. Immunocompromised patients admitted to health care facilities have an increased risk of being exposed to strains of multidrug-resistant *Staphylococcus aureus* (MRSA) and therefore are more difficult to treat. (127)

_____ 3. One exception to the self-limiting nature of viral infection is acquired immunodeficiency syndrome (AIDS). (128)

_____ 4. Protozoa are responsible for valley fever and histoplasmosis, a systemic fungal respiratory disease. (128)

_____ 5. An accidental needlestick is an example of portal of exit in the chain of infection. (126)

_____ 6. Microorganisms are present only in susceptible hosts. (129)

_____ 7. Health care–associated infections (HAIs) are most commonly transmitted by direct contact between health care workers and patients or from patient to patient. (131)

_____ 8. HIV is the most commonly transmitted infection by contaminated needles. (132)

_____ 9. JCAHO provides guidelines for transmission-based precautions in hospitals. (133)

_____ 10. The intact multilayered mucosa is the body's first line of defense against infection. (130)

SHORT ANSWER

Directions: Using your own words, answer each question in the space provided.

11. Identify five major classifications of pathogens and one example of a microorganism for each. (Table 9-1)

_____

_____

_____

12. Discuss disinfection and nursing implications for using disinfectants. (150)_____

_____

_____

_____

13. Identify at least five guidelines for Standard Precautions. (Box 9-4)_____

_____

_____

_____

14. What is the proper method for disposal of sharps? (Box 9-4)_____

_____

_____

15. Describe the procedure for gowning for contact isolation. *(Procedure 9-3)*_____

_____

_____

_____

31

16. Review the following nursing tasks and identify whether medical asepsis (MA) or surgical asepsis (SA) is necessary to prevent the spread of infection. Label each task as MA or SA. (126, 143)

_____ a. Assisting patient with meal tray
_____ b. Helping patient brush teeth
_____ c. Obtaining a urine specimen from an existing catheter
_____ d. Obtaining a throat swab for a culture
_____ e. Inserting a urinary catheter
_____ f. Changing the bed linens
_____ g. Replacing a colostomy bag
_____ h. Drawing up medication in a syringe
_____ i. Removing medication from a bubble pack
_____ j. Dressing change of a new surgical incision
_____ k. Suctioning the lower airway
_____ l. Suctioning the oral cavity

17. Place the steps of opening a wrapped sterile package in the correct order. (Box 9–10)

_____ Grasp the outer surface of the last and innermost flap; pull the flap back, allowing it to fall flat.
_____ Place the wrapped sterile package flat in the center of the work surface.
_____ Grasp the outside surface of the first side flap; open the side flap, allow it to lie flat on the table surface.
_____ Grasp the outer surface of the tip of the outermost flap; open the outer flap away from your body.
_____ Grasp the outside surface of the second side flap and allow it to lie flat on the table surface.
_____ Remove the tape or seal indicating the sterilization date.
_____ Perform hand hygiene.

MULTIPLE CHOICE

Directions: Select the best answer(s) for each of the following questions.

18. The patient has a large midline abdominal incision. With the specific purpose of reducing a possible reservoir of infection, the patient care technician: (128)
    1. wears gloves and mask at all times.
    2. isolates the patient's personal articles.
    3. has the patient cover mouth and nose when coughing.
    4. changes the dressing when it becomes soiled.

19. A patient with rubella needs to be transported to the X-ray department. What should the patient care technician do to prepare the patient for transport? (Box 9-8, Figure 9-6)
    1. Advise the patient to immediately wash hands after returning from the procedure.
    2. Call the X-ray department and inform them to wear gloves at all times.
    3. Dress the patient in an isolation gown and then apply a mask.
    4. Instruct the patient to wear a mask and follow cough etiquette.

20. When caring for a patient with tuberculosis who is on airborne precautions, the patient care technician should routinely use: (Box 9-8)
    1. regular mask and eyewear.
    2. gown and gloves.
    3. surgical handwashing and gloves.
    4. particulate respirator mask.

21. The patient care technician is aware that the body has normal defenses against infection. One of the defense mechanisms is an acidic environment. Which medication can affect the acidic environment? (Table 9-2)
    1. ciprofloxacin (Cipro)
    2. aluminum/magnesium antacid (Mylanta)
    3. doxycycline (Vibramycin)
    4. chlorhexidine gluconate (Hibiclens)

22. What is a rationale for the consistent use of Standard Precautions? (133)
    1. CDC recommends that health care workers use "universal blood and body fluid precautions."
    2. It is difficult to accurately identify all patients infected with blood-borne pathogens.
    3. Studies show that infection rates are unaffected by use of protective measures.
    4. Hand hygiene, gloves, masks, eye protection, and gowns are appropriate for patient contact.

23. Which patient needs to be placed into contact precautions? (Box 9-8)
    1. One who has a draining wound colonized with multidrug-resistant bacteria
    2. One who has cancer and is currently leukopenic
    3. One who has meningitis caused by invasive *Neisseria meningitidis*
    4. One who has tuberculosis caused by *Mycobacterium tuberculosis*

24. With which patient might you have the most difficulty maintaining a sterile technique throughout the procedure? (Box 9-9)
    1. 4-month-old infant who is crying and upset, but needs routine immunization
    2. 30-year-old woman who is obese and confused needs a Foley catheter inserted
    3. 50-year-old man is continuously coughing and needs a dressing change on upper chest
    4. 15-year-old cheerful patient with Down syndrome "wants to help" insert the IV

25. A patient who is HIV-positive and ready for discharge expresses fears about exposure of other family members, particularly young children, to the disease. What is the best response to help decrease the patient's fears and concerns? (130–131)
    1. Review general principles of infection control in the home setting.
    2. Review principles of mode of transmission for HIV.
    3. Encourage expression of fears and concerns and validate feelings.
    4. Suggest that the patient maintain contact with family using phone calls, email, or video conferencing.

26. The new patient care technician observes a health care provider who routinely comes out of a patient's room, goes to the sink, quickly soaps her hands, rinses, and then shakes water from her hands so that it splashes on the floor, sink, and her uniform. What should the new patient care technician do? (Box 9-8)
    1. Contact the infection-control nurse for advice.
    2. Do nothing because the health care provider is not accountable to the patient care technician.
    3. Check on the patient's status and then write up an incident report.
    4. Offer the health care provider a paper towel and assess understanding of hand hygiene.

27. Which patient is most likely to be susceptible to infection because of factors affecting immunologic defense mechanisms? (Box 9-2)
    1. A 5-year-old child who is not up to date on school immunizations
    2. A 35-year-old woman who has recently returned from Japan
    3. A 73-year-old man who recently had chemotherapy and radiation treatments
    4. A 55-year-old man who has a high-stress job and is overweight

CRITICAL THINKING ACTIVITIES

28. The patient care technician is caring for several patients. The patients include a frail 87-year-old woman with a hip fracture; a 78-year-old woman with advanced Alzheimer's who is being treated for dehydration secondary to incontinence of watery diarrhea, and a 60-year-old man who sustained a small perforation during a routine colonoscopy, which was recommended as part of his annual physical examination.
    a. Explain conditions that promote the onset of healthcare-associated infections (HAIs) for these patients. (131–132)_____
    _____
    _____

    b. What measures can be used to prevent HAIs? (131)
    _____
    _____
    _____
    _____
    _____

c. Although the health care provider has not currently ordered isolation precautions for any of these patients, the patient care technician should consider initiating isolation precautions for which patient? Identify the type of isolation that the patient care technician would choose and give the rationale that supports the decision. (Box 9-8)

_____

_____

_____

29. The patient care technician is caring for a 35-year-old patient who sustained a penetrating abdominal wound and multiple bruises and contusions in a farming accident. The abdominal wound was very contaminated, but cleaned before and during surgery. The wound-care specialist has been consulted and has taught the nursing staff how to do the dressing changes. The patient has a peripheral IV and is receiving IV antibiotics and pain medication. The patient care technician identifies that the patient is at risk for infection.

a. Give examples of questions that the patient care technician could use to collect data about factors that would affect the patient's immunologic defense mechanisms. (Box 9-2, Table 9-2)

_____

_____

_____

b. Explain why this patient is likely to have an inflammatory response and describe the physiologic process that will occur. (Box 9-2, Table 9-2)

_____

_____

_____

c. Describe the signs and symptoms that would occur if the patient developed a localized infection at the abdominal wound site or at the IV site. (131)

_____

_____

d. Describe the signs and symptoms that the patient care technician would be alert for that would signal a systemic infection. (131)

_____

_____

_____

10 Workplace Safety and Body Mechanics

FILL IN THE BLANK SENTENCES

Directions: For each abbreviation, write out the full term or phrase.

1. RACE:_____(156)
2. CDC:_____(152–153)
3. OSHA:_____(152)
4. PASS:_____(156)
5. NIOSH:_____(152)

TRUE OR FALSE

Directions: Write T for true or F for false in the blanks provided.

_____ 6. Fire prevention includes good housekeeping, maintenance, the elimination of all combustible material, and employee discipline. (Box 10.4)

_____ 7. Electrical accidents can be prevented by reporting frayed or broken electrical cords or any shocks felt when using equipment. (156)

_____ 8. The first action recommended in the event of ingestion of a poison is to use ipecac. (Injury & Illness Prevention Box 10.2)

_____ 9. The vast majority of occupational injuries requiring days away from work are classified as musculoskeletal disorders. (159)

_____ 10. Workplace violence is always physical. (Box 10.1)

MULTIPLE CHOICE

Directions: Select the best answer(s) for each of the following questions.

11. What is the rationale for flexing knees and keeping the feet shoulder-width apart when lifting a patient? (Table 10.1)
    1. Increases stability
    2. Keeps workload to a minimum
    3. Divides the workload by 50%
    4. Reduces risk of injury to the patient

12. What is the rationale for using a pull sheet when moving a patient? (Table 10.1)
    1. Increases stability
    2. Keeps workload to a minimum
    3. Divides the workload by 50%
    4. Reduces risk of injury to the patient

13. Disaster drills are part of which disaster planning intervention? (Box 10.5)
    1. Planning
    2. Evaluation
    3. Development
    4. Implementation

14. Which agency provides guidelines for violence identification and prevention programs? (Box 10.1)
    1. OSHA
    2. JCAHO
    3. CDC
    4. NIOSH

15. The patient care technician is reviewing the disaster preparedness plan for a small nursing home. What should be included in the plan? *(Select all that apply.)* (Box 10.6)
    1. Emergency treatment for the most critically injured
    2. Possible admission to a hospital or transfer to a temporary shelter
    3. Log to document residents' names and locations
    4. System to notify families and health care providers
    5. Designation of an area for decontamination
    6. Method of patient identification, such as a bracelet or picture ID

SHORT ANSWER

Directions: Using your own words, answer each question in the space provided.

16. Describe the risk factors contributing to workplace violence. (Box 10.1)_____

_____

_____

17. Describe the responsibilities of the patient care technician as they relate to fire prevention. (Box 10.4)_____

_____

_____

CRITICAL THINKING ACTIVITIES

Directions: Using your own words, answer each question in the space provided.

18. The patient care technician is working in a small urban outpatient clinic. The nurse manager has just informed the staff that the disaster plan may have to be activated because the emergency department of a nearby hospital has identified a possible bioterrorism-related event.
    a. What is the role of the patient care technician in a disaster event? (157–158, Box 10.5)_____

    _____

    _____

    b. How should the patient care technician prepare for a possible bioterrorism-related event in the workplace? (158)

    _____

    _____

19. List your personal fears or concerns about safety for family, friends, and self that might occur during a bioterrorism event. Discuss these fears and concerns with a classmate or your instructor.

_____

_____

_____

_____

11 Patient Safety

TRUE OR FALSE

Directions: Write T for true or F for false in the blanks provided.

_____1. A sentinel event is any unexpected occurrence involving death or serious physical or psychological injury, or the risk thereof. (162)

_____2. Errors do not need to be documented as long as they are corrected. (Delegation and Documentation Box 11.1)

_____3. A written order by the physician must detail the duration and circumstances under which safety reminder devices (SRDs) are to be used. (Box 11.4)

_____4. SRDs are primarily used in long-term care facilities. (164)

_____5. Radiation and radioactive materials are used in the diagnosis and treatment of patients. (166)

_____6. Items such as books, magazines, and shoes may be hazards that could cause the patient to fall. (Box 11.1)

ORDERING

7. Directions: In the blanks provided, identify the order of a mercury spill cleanup procedure. (Box 11.5)

_____ Dispose of collected mercury according to local environmental safety regulations.

_____ Evacuate the room except for a housekeeping crew (if available).

_____ Mop the floor with a mercury-specific cleanser (see agency policy).

_____ Ventilate the area. Close interior doors and open any outside windows.

FILL IN THE BLANK SENTENCES

Directions: Complete each sentence by filling in the blank with the correct word or phrase.

8. The focus on a safe environment has expanded to include _____ that come in contact with patients. (162)

9. Examples of _____ include medication errors and errors in procedures and treatments that led to the death of an individual and inappropriate application of safety reminder devices. (162)

10. According to OBRA, all other interventions should be attempted _____ the use of restraints. (Box 11.4)

11. Sources of mercury exposure in health care facilities include _____ and sphygmomanometers (blood pressure device). (166)

12. No one younger than _____ of age or who is or may be pregnant may visit someone receiving internal radiation therapy. (166)

13. The _____ applies SRDs and removes SRDs. (164)

MULTIPLE CHOICE

Directions: Select the best answer(s) for each of the following questions.

14. A safe environment implies freedom from injury with a focus on: (162)
    1. falls, electrical injuries, fires, burns, and poisoning.
    2. falls, workplace violence, fires, burns, and poisoning.
    3. falls, electrical injuries, fires, burns, and medication errors.
    4. falls, workplace violence, fires, burns, and medication errors.

15. A patient's fall risk assessment is completed: (162)
    1. upon discharge.
    2. when there is a staffing change.
    3. whenever the patient has a medical procedure.
    4. whenever there's a significant change in the patient's condition.

16. A policy which requires that every patient be evaluated on admission to determine the degree of likelihood for a potential fall is called: (Box 11.1)
    1. intake.
    2. triage.
    3. a fall precaution.
    4. a safety assessment.

17. The patient is using an older thermometer at home that contains mercury. The thermometer is dropped and breaks, releasing mercury onto the floor. What is the priority action? (Box 11.5)
    1. Evacuate everyone from the room.
    2. Close the interior doors and open windows.
    3. Vacuum the mercury and the glass shards.
    4. Mop the floor with hot water and soap.

18. Which occurrence is mostly likely to be investigated as a "sentinel event"? (162)
    1. Patient leaves the hospital against medical advice because she gets angry with the patient care technician.
    2. An older patient sustains a broken arm related to the use of an SRD.
    3. A patient receives his routine scheduled medication 2 hours late.
    4. During a follow-up phone call, a patient reports that care in the hospital was poor.

19. The patient care technician is observing the nurse conducting a fall risk assessment on an elderly patient who is moving into an assisted-living center. Which question(s) does the patient care technician expect the nurse to ask? (*Select all that apply.*) (Box 11.2)
    1. Have you had any falls in the past year?
    2. Are you able to independently get up after a fall?
    3. Do you feel unsteady when you stand up?
    4. Are you able to independently walk from room to room?
    5. Have you ever lost consciousness after a fall?
    6. Do you use a cane or other assistive device?

20. For the care of a patient who has an SRD in place, which task can be delegated to unlicensed assistive personnel (UAP)? (Delegation and Documentation Box 11.2)
    1. Observe for circulation distal to the SRD.
    2. Check for respiratory effort and breathing.
    3. Provide range-of-motion exercises.
    4. Determine when the SRD can be removed.

21. Which instructions should be given to the UAP who is assigned to assist in the care of a patient who is being treated with internal radiation? (166)
    1. Do not go into the room unless the patient uses the call bell.
    2. Help children don a lead shield apron before entering the room.
    3. Wear a mask, eye shield, and isolation gown when entering the room.
    4. Wear a device to record radiation exposure during patient care or when handling patient items.

22. The patient care technician is talking to a young mother who has an infant who has just started to crawl. Based on knowledge of growth and development, which safety issue is currently the most important to discuss with the mother? (163)
    1. What to do when using pots and pans on the stove
    2. How to ensure backyard pool safety measures
    3. How to manage electrical sockets and cords
    4. Where to obtain safety labels for cleaning products

23. Which of the following changes creates the greatest risk for falls for an older adult? (Injury & Illness Prevention Box 11.1)
    1. Vision changes
    2. Sensory overload
    3. Hearing changes
    4. Peripheral vascular system changes

Directions: Using your own words, answer each question in the space provided.

24. How can the patient care technician reduce his or her exposure to radiation? (166)

_____

_____

_____

25. Describe the ways in which the patient care technician can design a restraint-free environment. (Box 11.3)

_____

_____

_____

_____

26. Describe the impact the Omnibus Budget Reconciliation Act (OBRA) of 1987 had on SRDs. (Box 11.4)

_____

_____

_____

_____

12 Moving, Positioning, and Preventing Falls

WORD SCRAMBLE

Directions: Unscramble the words that describe different joint movements and then match the term to the correct definition. (Table 12.2)

Scrambled Term	Unscrambled Term	Definition
3. ynsperoexhtein		
4. bounctdia		
5. dodctianu		
6. nupsintioa		
7. raopntoni		
8. oorsidlexfin		

Definition of joint movements

a. Movement of limb away from body
b. The action of bending or the condition of being bent, especially the bending of a limb or joint
c. Kind of rotation that allows palm of hand to turn downward
d. To bend or flex backward
e. Movement of certain joints that decreases the angle between two adjoining bones
f. Movement of limb toward axis of body
g. Kind of rotation that allows palm of hand to turn upwards
h. Extreme or abnormal extension

MATCHING

Directions: Match the device on the left to the correct purpose on the right. (Table 12.1)

Device	Purpose
_____ 9. trochanter roll _____ 10. bed board _____ 11. side rail _____ 12. wedge pillow _____ 13. foot boots _____ 14. pillow _____ 15. hand-wrist splint _____ 16. sandbag	a. Helps weak patient to roll from side to side or to sit up in bed b. Used to maintain the legs in abduction after total hip replacement surgery c. Maintain feet in dorsiflexion, which prevents plantar flexion d. Provides support and shape to body contours; immobilizes extremity; maintains specific body alignment e. Individually molded for patient to maintain proper alignment of thumb; slightly adducted in opposition to fingers; maintains wrist in slight dorsiflexion f. Prevents external rotation of legs when patient is in supine position; possible to make with a bath blanket g. Provides support of body or extremity; elevates body part; splints incisional area to reduce postoperative pain during activity or coughing and deep-breathing h. Provides additional support to mattress and improves vertebral alignment

FILL IN THE BLANK SENTENCES

Directions: Complete each sentence by filling in the blank with the correct word or phrase.

17. When using hydraulic lifts for transfers of older adults, particularly for those with _____, it is reassuring to provide basic instructions and make sure they have their eyeglasses (if they use them). (*Injury and Illness Prevention* Box 12.1)

18. Use a(n) _____ to assist with ambulation for patients with continuous IV therapy. (*Delegation and Documentation Box 12.1*)

19. Muscles decrease in size and _____ when not continually used. (Box 12.1)

TRUE OR FALSE

Directions: Write T for true or F for false in the blanks provided.

_____ 20. Weakness and low blood pressure are common signs and symptoms noted in an older adult on bedrest. (Injury and Illness Prevention Box 12.1)

_____ 21. Safety reminder devices are primarily used to keep staff safe. (182)

_____ 22. Immobility always results from trauma. (188)

SHORT ANSWER

Directions: Using your own words, answer each question in the space provided.

23. Describe several body mechanics and positioning techniques that protect the patient care technician from physical injury. (*Procedure 12.3*)

_____

_____

_____

24. Discuss why impaired mobility may lead to depression, agitation, or emotional distress. (Box 12.1)

_____

_____

_____

MULTIPLE CHOICE

Directions: Select the best answer(s) for each of the following questions.

25. Which of the following assistive devices can be used to immobilize an extremity when a patient needs prolonged bed rest? (Table 12.1)
    1. Pillow
    2. Side rail
    3. Sandbag
    4. Bed board

26. The patient experienced a cerebrovascular accident (CVA) that left her with severe left-sided paralysis and very limited mobility. Which device would prevent plantar flexion? (Table 12.1)
    1. Footboard
    2. Bed board
    3. Trapeze bar
    4. Trochanter roll

27. Which patient has a contracture? (*Procedure 12.2*)
    1. Patient has abnormal extension of a finger joint.
    2. Patient's wrist is abnormally flexed and joint is fixed.
    3. Patient's knee is hyperextended.
    4. Patient has abnormal lateral movements of ankle joint.

28. What is the most likely complication if an elderly patient gets pulled across the bed when changing wet linens? (Injury and Illness Prevention Box 12.1)
    1. Dislocation of a joint
    2. Increased stress to the joints
    3. Abnormal hyperextension of a joint
    4. Shearing or tearing of the skin

29. For an older female patient who is at risk for osteoporosis, which associated complication can be minimized by participating in a regular exercise program as prescribed by the health care provider? (Injury & Illness Prevention Box 12.1)
    1. Bone loss that results in fractures
    2. Immobility secondary to joint degeneration
    3. Tissue ischemia and pressure ulcers
    4. Thrombophlebitis secondary to blood clots

30. Which of the following is a complication of immobility? (Box 12.1)
    1. Diarrhea
    2. Dehydration
    3. Kidney stones
    4. Increased fatigue

CRITICAL THINKING ACTIVITIES

Directions: Using your own words, answer each question in the space provided.

31. The patient care technician is caring for a patient who has had a CVA with right-sided impairment. The patient has difficulty moving her right arm and leg and this results in interference with activities of daily living (ADLs).
    a. Before turning or transferring this patient, what patient assessment and preparations should be made? (*Procedure 12.3*)

    _____

    _____

    b. Identify the appropriate action to assist the patient to move from the bed to a chair. (*Procedure 12.3*)

    _____

    _____

    c. While transferring the patient from the bed to a chair, the patient starts to fall. What should the patient care technician do? (*Procedure 12.6*)

    _____

    _____

    d. The patient is unable to perform range of motion (ROM) of the right extremities. What can the patient care technician do to help the patient accomplish the ROM exercises? (Table 12.2)

    _____

    _____

32. The patient care technician is caring for a patient who is in a comatose state after sustaining a severe head injury several months ago. He is breathing on his own and his vital signs are stable but he shows no purposeful movements.
    a. What are the complications of immobility for this patient? (Box 12.1)_____

    _____

b. What interventions may be implemented to prevent the occurrence of complications of immobility? (Box 12.1, Table 12.1)

_____

_____

_____

13 Basic Emergency Care

VOCABULARY REVIEW

Directions: Define the following terms.

1. Cyanosis: (195)_____

_____

2. Idiopathic: (197)_____

_____

3. Abrasion: (198)_____

_____

4. Fibrillation: (191)_____

_____

5. Myocardium: (191)_____

_____

6. Asystole: (189)_____

_____

FILL IN THE BLANK SENTENCES

Directions: Fill in the blanks with the correct terms.

7. _____ is defined as the immediate care given to a person who has been injured or has suddenly become ill. (189)

8. AED stands for _____. (189)

9. CPR stands for _____. (189)

10. The goal of the _____ is to respond when a patient is rapidly declining so they may be able to prevent the patient from getting worse than he or she already is, or even death. (190)

11. A(n) _____ is transient and occurs with a rapid rise in body temperature over 101.8 ° F (38.8 ° C). (197)

12. Start CPR if a child's heart rate is fewer than _____ per minute. (*Procedure 13.3*)

Directions: Read the case studies and answer the questions that follow.

13. A 19-year-old patient sitting in the waiting room experiences a grand mal seizure. What should Cheryl, the patient care technician, do to prevent injury to the patient? After the seizure, the patient needs to be placed in the recovery position to maintain her airway. Explain how to place her in this position. (197)

_____

_____

_____

14. The mother of a 10-year-old child comes running into the office with her son. He is bleeding profusely from a gash in his left forearm. She states he fell on some glass at the playground and she just rushed him to the physician's office. What should be done immediately to control the bleeding from the wound? (198–199; *Procedure 13.5*)

_____

_____

_____

15. A patient complains of feeling dizzy and faint when the patient care technician enters the room. While inquiring about the patient's symptoms, the patient suddenly faints. What should the patient care technician have done when the patient complained of dizziness? What should the technician do after the patient had fainted? (192–194; *Procedure 13.2*)

_____

_____

_____

MULTIPLE CHOICE

Directions: Select the best answer(s) for each of the following questions.

16. Which meets the criteria for calling the Rapid Response Team? (*Select all that apply.*) (Table 13.1)
    1. Intense pain
    2. Sudden change in mental status
    3. Respiratory rate over 28/min or fewer than 8/min
    4. Heart rate over 140/min or fewer than 60/min
    5. Potential for obstructed airway

17. A closed wound with no evidence of injury to the skin describes a(n): (198)
    1. contusion.
    2. abrasion.
    3. avulsion.
    4. puncture.

18. What is the best course of action for an object lodged in body tissues? (198)
    1. Leave it there.
    2. Apply pressure.
    3. Remove immediately.
    4. Cover with sterile dressing.

19. Complete or partial removal of a finger is an example of a(n): (198)
    1. contusion.
    2. abrasion.
    3. avulsion.
    4. puncture.

20. Which is a sign of an open airway? (194)
    1. Rising chest
    2. Rapid breaths
    3. Consciousness
    4. Patient talking

SHORT ANSWER

Directions: Using your own words, answer each question in the space provided.

21. Cheryl is in charge of assembling the office crash cart. What types of supplies should be stocked in the cart? What medications should be included? How should the cart and supplies be maintained? Where should the cart be kept? (190, Box 13.1)

    _____

    _____

    _____

    _____

    _____

22. The patient care technician can play an integral role in a community's response to natural or human-created disasters. Summarize how the technician can contribute to the community response to an emergency. (200)

    _____

    _____

    _____

    _____

23. The daughter of an elderly stroke victim is very concerned about her father's potential for choking. Explain to the daughter what to do if her father experiences an obstructed airway. Include in your explanation the techniques for both responsive and unresponsive adults. (*Procedure 13.4*)

    _____

    _____

    _____

    _____

14 Assisting with the Physical Examination

MATCHING

Match the following terms with their definitions.

Term	Definition
_____ 1. bruit (203)	a. Abnormal sound or murmur heard on auscultation
_____ 2. gait (203)	b. White part of the eye
_____ 3. clubbing (211)	c. Movement of the body by applied force
_____ 4. transillumination (211)	d. Physical injury caused by an external force or violence
_____ 5. trauma (203)	e. Style of walking
_____ 6. sclera (211)	f. Inspection of a cavity or organ by passing light through its walls
_____ 7. manipulation (213)	g. The use of touch during the physical examination to assess the size, consistency, and location of certain body parts
_____ 8. palpation (207)	h. Abnormal enlargement of the distal phalanges associated with cyanotic heart disease or advanced chronic pulmonary disease

FILL IN THE BLANK SENTENCES

Directions: Fill in the blanks with the correct vocabulary terms from the chapter.

9. _____ describes the act of listening to body sounds to assess various organs throughout the body. (207)

10. Brain lesions can cause _____, which manifests as a lack of coordination and failure to arrange words in proper order. (211)

11. A faulty heart valve creates a(n) _____. (207)

12. A(n) _____ is a small lump, lesion, or swelling felt when the skin is palpated. (211)

13. A(n) _____ is an abnormal sound auscultated over a blood vessel. (203)

14. In a(n) _____ procedure, the physician uses a fiberoptic instrument to view the inside of the large intestine. (203)

SHORT ANSWER

Directions: Using your own words, answer each question in the space provided.

15. Summarize the major guidelines for proper body mechanics. (213)_____

_____

_____

_____

_____

16. Describe how to transfer a patient safely from a wheelchair to the examination table. (209)

_____

_____

_____

_____

17. Describe the typical physical examination sequence. (210–212)_____

_____

_____

_____

_____

MULTIPLE CHOICE

Directions: Select the best answer(s) for each of the following questions.

18. Which statement is an accurate description of the hospitalist? (203)
    1. Present in outpatient facilities only
    2. Collaborate with the primary care physician
    3. Only available during peak times
    4. Represent a particular physician's office

19. Which are acceptable patient identifiers? (*Select all that apply.*) (204)
    1. Room number
    2. Patient's name
    3. Date of birth
    4. Physical location
    5. Allergies

20. Which are patient preparation tasks that should always be performed by the patient care technician? (*Select all that apply.*) (204–205)
    1. Obtain signatures for consents.
    2. Place patient records in the designated area.
    3. Obtain a urine sample for all female patients.
    4. Help the patient physically prepare for the examination.
    5. Measure and record the patient's height, weight, body mass index, and vital signs.

21. Which is an accurate statement about the physical examination? (205)
    1. Can be delegated to the patient care technician
    2. Equipment should be retrieved as needed
    3. Performed from the feet to the head
    4. Performed from the head to the feet

22. Which physical examination method ranges from focusing on the patient's general appearance to more detailed observations? (207)
    1. Inspection
    2. Palpation
    3. Percussion
    4. Mensuration

23. A sclera with a yellow tone is indicative of which condition? (211)
    1. Lung disease
    2. Renal disease
    3. Liver disease
    4. Diabetes

Measuring and Recording Vital Signs

MATCHING

Directions: Match the following terms with their definitions.

Definition	Term
_____ 1. An individual must sit or stand to breathe comfortably	a. arrhythmia (225)
_____ 2. Fever	b. rales (215)
_____ 3. A brief lapse in consciousness	c. pyrexia (217)
_____ 4. Pulse that is thready or bounding	d. tachypnea (215)
_____ 5. A continuous, dry rattling in the throat or bronchial tube caused by partial obstruction	e. rhonchi (215)
_____ 6. Crackling breath sounds during inspiration	f. orthopnea (227)
_____ 7. Condition marked by rapid, shallow respirations	g. bradypnea (215)
_____ 8. Respirations that are regular in rhythm but slower than normal in rate	h. syncope (215)
_____ 9. Absence or cessation of breathing	i. stertorous (215)
_____ 10. A strenuous respiratory effort marked by a snoring sound	j. apnea (215)

TRUE OR FALSE

Directions: Indicate which statements are true (T) and which are false (F).

_____ 11. A change in one or more of the patient's vital signs may indicate a change in general health. (216)

_____ 12. Sometimes vital sign measurements must be obtained a second time after the patient is calmer or more comfortable. (216)

_____ 13. Body temperature is regulated by the hypothalamus. (216)

_____ 14. Body temperature ranges from being highest in the morning to being lowest in the late afternoon. (216)

_____ 15. Patients with a febrile condition exhibit pyrexia and can be treated with an antipyretic. (217)

_____ 16. An individual with hypertension may have a bounding pulse. (228)

_____ 17. A contraindication for taking a temporal artery temperature is bilateral impacted cerumen. (219)

_____ 18. Primary or essential hypertension is idiopathic. (228)

_____ 19. The difference between tachypnea and hyperpnea is that respirations are rapid and shallow with hyperpnea. (215)

_____ 20. Otitis externa is known as "swimmer's ear." (215)

_____ 21. Frequent spirometer studies will be ordered for a patient diagnosed with chronic obstructive pulmonary disease (COPD) to determine the person's breathing capabilities. (227)

_____ 22. Secondary hypertension is caused by another underlying pathologic condition. (228)

SHORT ANSWER

Directions: Using your own words, answer each question in the space provided.

23. Summarize the American Heart Association's recommendations for the prevention and treatment of hypertension. (228–229)

_____

_____

24. List and define the five Korotkoff phases. (231–232) _____

_____

_____

_____

_____

25. Explain four common causes of errors in blood pressure readings. (Box 15.3) _____

_____

_____

_____

26. List and describe three factors that may affect body temperature. (216) _____

_____

_____

_____

MULTIPLE CHOICE

Directions: Select the best answer(s) for each of the following questions.

27. Which is a cardinal vital sign? (*Select all that apply.*) (216)
    1. Pain
    2. Weight
    3. Respiratory rate
    4. Fat composition

28. A fever that comes and goes, or spikes and then returns to the average range, is called: (217)
    1. axillary.
    2. remittent.
    3. continuous.
    4. intermittent.

29. Which thermometer type should not be used in a health care setting? (222)
    1. Axillary
    2. Disposable
    3. Tympanic
    4. Temporal artery scanner

30. Which pulse site is best found on the thumb side of the wrist, 1 inch below the base of the thumb? (224)
    1. Radial
    2. Apical
    3. Brachial
    4. Femoral

31. A patient with a significant difference between the apical and brachial pulse counts has: (223)
    1. bradycardia.
    2. a pulse deficit.
    3. an intermittent pulse.
    4. tachycardia.

32. The amount of blood in the arteries is called: (228)
    1. pulse.
    2. volume.
    3. vessel elasticity.
    4. blood viscosity.

16 Obtaining and Monitoring an Electrocardiogram

MATCHING

Directions: Match the following terms with their definitions.

Term	Definition
_____ 1. bradycardia (241)	a. Result of the absence of a heartbeat or cardiac cessation
_____ 2. bundle of His (241)	b. A procedure used for the diagnosis of heart disease
_____ 3. asystole (253)	c. An irregular heart rhythm
_____ 4. electrocardiography (240)	d. A heart rate of fewer than 60 beats per minute
_____ 5. V-fib (253)	e. Fibers that conduct electrical impulses from the atrioventricular node (AV) node to the ventricular myocardium
_____ 6. electrode (244)	f. Placed on the patient's arms, legs, and chest to pick up the electrical activity of the heart
_____ 7. myocardial (240)	g. Pertaining to the heart muscle
_____ 8. arrhythmia (241)	h. Occurs when the electrical conduction system of the heart is in total dysfunction

FILL IN THE BLANK SENTENCES

Directions: Complete each sentence by filling in the blank with the correct word or phrase.

9. The _____ are the two upper chambers of the heart. (240)

10. The _____ are the two lower chambers of the heart. (240)

11. _____ is the medical term for the heart muscle. (241)

12. The _____ node controls the rate of heart contractions by initiating electrical impulses 60 to 100 times per minute. (241)

13. The first three leads recorded in an electrocardiogram (ECG) are called the _____ or _____ leads because each lead uses two limb electrodes to record the heart's electrical activity. (244)

14. The electrical activity recorded by the three _____ leads is relatively small so the ECG machine amplifies the electrical activity of each to record them on the strip. (244–245)

15. One millivolt of electrical activity moves the stylus upward over _____. (244)

16. The _____ wave occurs during the contraction of the atria and shows the beginning of cardiac depolarization. (243)

17. The _____ complex shows the contraction of both ventricles and also reflects the completion of cardiac depolarization. (243)

18. The _____ interval is the time from the beginning of atrial contraction to the beginning of ventricular contraction. (243)

19. The T wave indicates ventricular recovery, or _____ of the ventricles. (243)

20. ECG paper has horizontal and vertical lines at _____ -mm intervals. (243)

21. When running at normal speed, one small, 1-mm square passes the stylus every _____ seconds. (244)

22. Lead I records the electrical activity between the _____ arm and the _____ arm. (244)

23. _____ records the electrical activity of the atria from the right shoulder. (245)

24. Describe diastole and systole. (241) _____

_____

_____

_____

_____

25. Describe the electrical conduction system of the heart. (241) _____

_____

_____

_____

_____

26. You have been instructed to perform an ECG on a 51-year-old man. As you start to prepare the patient for the examination, you notice a large amount of body hair on his chest. Can the procedure still be performed? What should you do? Why? (*Procedure 16.1*)

_____

_____

_____

MULTIPLE CHOICE

Directions: Select the best answer(s) for each of the following questions.

27. Which rhythm is shown in the illustration below? (251)

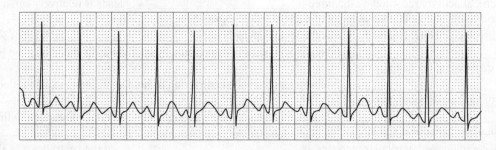

1. Sinus tachycardia
2. Sinus bradycardia
3. Ventricular tachycardia
4. Ventricular fibrillation

28. Which rhythm is shown in the illustration below? (241)

1. Sinus tachycardia
2. Normal sinus rhythm
3. Ventricular tachycardia
4. Ventricular fibrillation

29. The standard speed for an ECG recording is: (244)
1. 10 mm/sec.
2. 20 mm/sec.
3. 25 mm/sec.
4. 35 mm/sec.

30. During the ECG recording, the patient coughs and starts talking. What would you expect to see? (249)
1. Somatic tremor
2. Interrupted baseline
3. Wandering baseline
4. Alternating current interference

31. The likelihood of alternating current interference can be decreased by: (249)
1. keeping lead wires crossed.
2. moving the table against the wall.
3. instructing patient to remain still.
4. unplugging other electrical appliances in the room.

32. The physician has reviewed a patient's ECG and has concluded that the patient has premature atrial contractions (PACs). What could be the cause of the PACs? (251)
1. High stress levels
2. Blockage of the supplying artery
3. Patient moving or talking during the test
4. Consumption of large amounts of caffeine

Student Name_____ Date_____

 17 Assisting with Admissions and Discharge

FILL IN THE BLANK SENTENCES

Directions: Complete each sentence by filling in the blank with the correct word or phrase.

1. _____ addresses the patient's right to refuse or accept medical treatment, as well as information regarding advance directives. (259)
2. The _____, _____, and _____ require that all hospitals and other health care facilities present a Patient's Bill of Rights to the patient or the patient's legal guardian at the time of admission. (259)
3. An interagency transfer requires documentation from the _____ and the health care provider and a(n) _____ from the patient indicating that he or she understands the risks and benefits associated with the transfer. (626)
4. The Joint Commission (TJC) requires each hospitalized patient to have an admission assessment prepared by a registered nurse within _____ hour(s) of admission. (Box 17.1 Delegation and Documentation)

MULTIPLE CHOICE

Directions: Select the best answer(s) for each of the following questions.

5. During the admission of a patient to a health care facility, the responsibilities of the admission department representative include: (*Select all that apply.*) (258–259)
   1. obtaining identifying information.
   2. giving information on the Health Insurance Portability and Accountability Act.
   3. placing the correct ID band on the patient's wrist.
   4. obtaining a list of current medications.
   5. obtaining emergency contact information.
   6. gathering insurance information.

6. Which newly admitted patient is mostly likely to need and benefit from an individualized explanation of the bathroom facilities? (*Procedure 17.1*)
   1. A 75-year-old woman with advanced Alzheimer's disease
   2. A 20-month-old child who has just started toilet training
   3. A 65-year-old man who is from a rural farming region of China
   4. A 50-year-old woman who has stress incontinence

7. The patient care technician is placing an ID band on a patient who was admitted through the emergency department. What is the best thing to say as the band is applied? (258)
   1. "This is your assigned hospital identification number."
   2. "The primary purpose of the band is to maintain safety."
   3. "All patients have to wear these; it's standard procedure."
   4. "We don't want to lose you while you are in the hospital."

8. The patient is newly admitted and seems anxious, but also appears very tentative about asking questions. Which statement by the patient care technician best demonstrates empathy? (258)
   1. "Call me if you need anything; I'll be happy to help you."
   2. "There's nothing to worry about; we'll take good care of you."
   3. "I know you must have a lot of questions; I know I would."
   4. "You seem a little uncertain; do you have some questions?"

9. The patient care technician is trying to explain the bed controls and the call button and other items related to hospitalization, but the elderly patient keeps telling the patient care technician to "wait for my son to get here." What should the patient care technician do first? (*Procedure 17.1*)
   1. Go find the son or other available family members.
   2. Leave written information at the bedside.
   3. Give brief information using very simple language.
   4. Offer comfort measures and ensure patient safety.

57

Copyright © 2023 by Elsevier Inc. All rights reserved.

Chapter **17** Assisting with Admissions and Discharge

10. The patient tells the patient care technician that he would like to be transferred to hospital X, because his cardiologist doesn't come to hospital Y. What should the patient care technician do? (262)
    1. Obtain an Against Medical Advice form and have the patient sign it.
    2. Call hospital X and advise that the patient desires transfer.
    3. Advise the patient that the cardiologists in hospital Y are good.
    4. Advise the patient that a transfer requires an order from the health care provider and inform the nurse of the patient's request.
11. Which patient is likely to have the most complex discharge plan? (262–263)
    1. A 73-year-old man with chronic disease who has no family in the area
    2. A 23-year-old mother who just delivered her first healthy baby
    3. A 17-year-old adolescent who broke his leg during a ski trip
    4. A 35-year-old woman who had an emergency appendectomy

CRITICAL THINKING ACTIVITIES

12. Identify and record the patient's reaction to hospitalization in the blanks provided.
    a. Patient appears anxious as he enters his hospital room for the first time. He nervously begins to ask the patient care technician a series of questions about what will happen to him. Reaction: _____ (257)
    b. A preschooler who is admitted to the hospital is happily engaged in playing with the toys that the patient care technician has provided, but when her parents prepare to leave, she begins to cry and clings to them. Reaction: _____ (258)
    c. An elderly woman who has just moved into an assisted-living facility seems to need a lot of social interaction. She becomes very talkative when the patient care technician tries to leave the room. Reaction: _____ (258)
    d. An adolescent is admitted to the hospital, but refuses to take off his clothes and put on a hospital gown. Reaction: _____ (258)
13. The patient is admitted through the emergency department for an exacerbation of a chronic respiratory disorder. When the patient arrives to the room, he appears very tired. He has oxygen via nasal cannula and demonstrates labored breathing. He is able to speak, but his sentences are short and he takes a breath after every few words. How would the patient care technician modify the actions related to the admission to meet the needs of this patient? (Box 17.4)
    a. Checking and verifying ID band: _____

    _____

    b. Assessing immediate needs: _____

    _____

    c. Explaining hospital routines, such as visiting hours, mealtime, and morning wake-up: _____

    _____

    d. Orienting the patient to the room: _____

    _____

    _____

14. A 45-year-old woman was admitted to the hospital for chronic infection of a stasis ulcer on her leg. She will be discharged after completing antibiotic therapy and consultation with the wound care specialist.
    a. Identify examples of health care disciplines other than nursing that are involved in referrals, and explain their role in the discharge process. (*Injury and Illness Prevention* Box 17.1)

    _____

    _____

    _____

b. Provide the rationale for each of the following actions in the discharge of a patient. (*Procedure 17.3*)

   i. Makes certain there is a written discharge order: _____

_____

   ii. Notifies the family or person who will be transporting the patient home:_____

_____

   iii. Gathers equipment, supplies, and prescriptions that the patient is to take home:_____

_____

   iv. Assists the patient with dressing and packing items to go home: _____

_____

Chapter **17** **Assisting with Admissions and Discharge**

This page intentionally left blank

18 Bedmaking and Hygiene

TRUE OR FALSE

Directions: Write T for true or F for false in the blanks provided.

_____ 1. Baths rehydrate the older patient's skin. (269, Lifespan Considerations for Older Adults Box)

_____ 2. Urinary incontinence is expected among very elderly adults. (269, Lifespan Considerations for Older Adults Box)

_____ 3. Medicare and Medicaid will cover the costs of treating pressure ulcers that developed during the patient's hospitalization if the condition is well-documented. (277)

_____ 4. When the external pressure against the skin is greater than the pressure in the capillary bed, blood flow increases to the adjacent tissues. (277)

_____ 5. Routine hygiene would include trimming or shaving an unsightly beard, mustache, or sideburns for surgical procedures or to maintain personal cleanliness. (Box 18.4)

FILL IN THE BLANK SENTENCES

Directions: Complete each sentence by filling in the blank with the correct word or phrase.

6. Assisting a patient with hygiene gives the patient care technician an opportunity to assist the patient with the performance of _____. (267)

7. The recommended room temperature for most adult patients is _____. (269)

8. If external pressure on the skin or tissues continues without relief for more than _____ hours, cells in the involved layers of skin tend to undergo necrosis. (277)

9. Inserting objects into the internal auditory canal can damage the _____ or cause _____ to become impacted in the canal. (282)

10. The appearance of pressure ulcers is a major cause of impaired _____. (277)

MULTIPLE CHOICE

Directions: Select the best answer(s) for each of the following questions.

11. The nurse is teaching a patient who has diabetes about foot care. What does the patient care technician expect will be included in the patient's self-care instructions? (Box 18.2)
    1. Carefully cut corns and apply moleskin.
    2. Inspect feet daily for breaks in the skin.
    3. Wear loose shoes or sandals to air the feet.
    4. Use alcohol to increase dryness between the toes.

12. In delegating the early morning care that should occur before breakfast, what does the patient care technician remind the unlicensed assistive personnel (UAP) to do for the patient? (Box 18.3)
    1. Shampoo the patient's hair and comb it.
    2. Assist the patient with a bath and clean gown.
    3. Offer the patient a backrub with warmed lotion.
    4. Help the patient wash hands and face.

13. A patient who is paralyzed from the waist down is at risk for developing a pressure ulcer on the sacral area. Which intervention would be used for this patient? (277)
    1. Frequently check and change the bed linens.
    2. Teach to shift weight every 15 minutes.
    3. Obtain an order for a donut cushion for sitting.
    4. Keep skin moist and frequently reapply lotion.

14. While completing the bath, the patient care technician notices a reddened area on the patient's sacrum. What should the patient care technician do first? (*Injury and Illness Prevention* Box 18.1)
    1. Cleanse the skin with alcohol.

2. Wash the area with hot water and soap.
3. Massage the area vigorously.
4. Assess for other areas of erythema.

15. The patient care technician is evaluating the eye care that has been delegated to and is being provided by a new staff member. Which action is appropriate? (282)
1. Removing dried secretions with moist gauze
2. Using soap and water on a washcloth
3. Cleansing the eyes from the outer to the inner canthus
4. Wiping plastic eyeglasses with a clean paper towel

16. The patient care technician observes the patient performing ear care. Identify which behavior indicates a need for additional teaching. (*Delegation and Documentation* Box 18.2)
1. Cleans the pinna with a cotton-tipped swab
2. Turns the hearing aid off when not in use
3. Leaves the hearing aid by a sunny window
4. Rotates a clean washcloth to clean ear canal

17. The patient care technician is caring for a postpartum patient. Which assessment should the patient care technician perform first before starting perineal care? (*Procedure 18.2*)
1. Note presence of accumulated secretions.
2. Evaluate the appearance of episiotomy.
3. Assess ability to perform own care.
4. Ask about burning with urination.

18. The nurse is supervising a student patient care technician who is giving a patient a bed bath. The nurse would intervene if the student performed which action? (271)
1. Lowers the side rail to perform care
2. Raises the head of the bed to a semi-Fowler's position
3. Bathes arms using long, firm strokes
4. Puts up all four side rails after completing the bath

19. The nurse instructed the patient care technician to encourage the patient's independence in performing personal hygiene. Which behavior best indicates that the patient care technician understood what to do? (*Delegation and Documentation* Box 18.1)
1. The patient care technician waits until the patient uses the call light for assistance.
2. The nurse sees that the commode chair is close to the bed.
3. The nurse observes that the patient is brushing his own teeth.
4. The patient care technician tells the nurse that the patient is independent for ADLs.

CRITICAL THINKING ACTIVITY

20. For the following patients, identify how bathing may be affected or altered.
a. The patient has dementia. (Box 18-5) _____

_____

b. The patient is on complete bedrest. (*Procedure 18-1*) _____

_____

c. The patient has a hearing aid. (282) _____

_____

d. There is inflammation of the perineal tissue. (281) _____

_____

e. The patient is an East Indian Hindu. (Box 18.1) _____

_____

19 Assisting with Grooming

TRUE OR FALSE

Directions: Write T for true or F for false in the blanks provided.

_____ 1. Hand hygiene doesn't need to be performed prior to performing hair care. (*Procedure 19.1*)

_____ 2. Some facilities may not permit patient care technicians to trim the nails of diabetics. (*Procedure 19.3*)

_____ 3. All head coverings should be labeled with the patient's name. (*Injury and Illness Prevention* Box 19.1)

_____ 4. Dandruff presents as excessive flaking skin that is white in color and is highly contagious. (288)

_____ 5. A male patient's beard, mustache, or sideburns may only be removed without consent of the patient in emergency situations. (290)

FILL IN THE BLANK SENTENCES

Directions: Complete each sentence by filling in the blank with the correct word or phrase.

6. Use shaving cream or soap if a(n) _____ is not available. (*Procedure 19.2*)

7. Extended soaking of the feet should be avoided for _____ patients. (*Procedure 19.3*)

8. _____ is head lice. (289)

9. The patient care technician may notice signs of _____ on a patient undergoing chemotherapy. (288)

10. There is an increased risk of _____ when shaving someone with a razor blade. (290)

MULTIPLE CHOICE

Directions: Select the best answer(s) for each of the following questions.

11. The patient care technician is preparing to shampoo a patient's hair. The patient care technician notices that the patient's hair is matted with blood. What is the appropriate action? (*Procedure 19.1*)
    1. Use witch hazel to clean the hair.
    2. Use extra shampoo to clean the hair.
    3. Use extra-hot water to clean the hair.
    4. Use hydrogen peroxide to clean the hair.

12. Which is an accurate statement regarding shaving a patient? (*Procedure 19.2*)
    1. Always use shaving cream or soap.
    2. Dispose of blades in sharps container.
    3. Avoid using disposable razors on the face.
    4. Shave against the direction of hair growth.

13. The patient care technician is caring for a patient undergoing anticoagulant therapy. The patient care technician should avoid: (290)
    1. shampooing with warm or hot water.
    2. having the patient stand for extended periods.
    3. shaving the patient with a disposable razor.
    4. soaking the patient's feet for extended periods of time.

14. The patient care technician is brushing the patient's hair and notices a bald part of the scalp with flaking of the skin. What should the patent care technician do? (288–289)
    1. Shampoo with dandruff treatment.
    2. Rinse the scalp with cool water.
    3. Massage the area vigorously.
    4. Notify the nurse immediately.

15. The patient care technician is tending to a female patient who states, "No one cares about me." The patient laments that she has had no visitors. Which action might lift the patient's spirits? (290)
    1. Calling the patient's family
    2. Offering to paint her fingernails
    3. Reassuring the patient that she is cared for
    4. Telling the patient that she shouldn't dwell on negativity

Student Name_____ Date_____

 Assisting with Medication Administration

TRUE OR FALSE

Directions: Write T for true or F for false in the blanks provided.

_____ 1. In most acute-care facilities, the Patient Care Technician may assist the patient with administration of their prescribed medications. (297)

_____ 2. Asking family to keep original medication bottles with the labels intact can help prevent medication errors. (297)

_____ 3. The trade name of a drug is usually longer, may refer to the chemical composition of the medication, and is not capitalized. (298)

_____ 4. Evidence-based practice for patient to determine when the metered-dose inhaler (MDI) is empty is to float the MDI in water. (*Procedure 20.10: Administering Metered-Dose Inhaler*)

_____ 5. Verifying the medication order is the first step to administering any medication. (299)

FILL IN THE BLANK SENTENCES

Directions: Complete each sentence by filling in the blank with the correct word or phrase.

6. In the home setting, it is important to have the original bottle of medications so that you can verify the correct _____, _____ and _____. (297)

7. A _____ _____ is the ordered amount of medication that the patient is supposed to receive at a prescribed time. (297)

8. _____ requires testing for all approved medications. (298)

9. _____ is the use of excessive numbers of different medications. (309, Lifespan Considerations Box)

10. _____ tablets are encased by a coated shell that keeps the tablet from being absorbed in the stomach. (301)

SHORT ANSWER

Directions: Using your own words, answer each question in the space provided.

11. Describe ways the patient care technician can help prevent medication administration errors. (Box 20.3)

_____

_____

_____

_____

12. List the six "rights" of medication administration. (Box 20.1)

a. _____

b. _____

c. _____

d. _____

e. _____

f. _____

13. List the three label checks of medication administration. (Box 20.2)

a. _____

b. _____

c. _____

MULTIPLE CHOICE

Directions: Select the best answer(s) for each of the following questions.

14. Medication labels should include which of the following information? (*Select all that apply.*) (298)
    1. Patient's name
    2. Patient's date of birth
    3. Route of administration
    4. Dose size and frequency
    5. Health care provider's name

15. Which abbreviation means four times a day? (Table 20.1)
    1. ac
    2. bed
    3. qid
    4. tid

16. The sublingual medication administrations means that a medication is given: (304)
    1. orally.
    2. in the cheek.
    3. under the tongue.
    4. through the skin or mucus membranes.

17. Which of the following is a percutaneous medication administration route? (304)
    1. instillation
    2. intradermal
    3. intramuscular
    4. subcutaneous

18. Which of the following complicates medication administration in older adults? (*Select all that apply.*) (309, Lifespan Considerations Box)
    1. Dry mouth
    2. Polypharmacy
    3. Decreased patient compliance
    4. Diminished hearing and vision
    5. Reduced awareness and cognitive abilities

21 Assisting with Nutrition and Fluids

FILL IN THE BLANK SENTENCES

Directions: Complete each sentence by filling in the blank with the correct word or phrase.

1. Nutrition is the sum of all body processes involved in taking in _____ and using them to maintain body tissue and provide energy. (310)

2. _____ can help prevent complications resulting from an imbalance in fluid intake and output or in electrolyte concentration. (320)

3. Keeping the IV insertion site _____ reduces the possibility of infection. (322)

4. Soft diets often serve as an intermediate step when a patient is progressing from _____. (314)

5. _____ is a test used to check how well the kidneys are working. (320)

TRUE OR FALSE

Directions: Write T for true or F for false in the blanks provided.

_____ 6. The nurse may delegate to the PCT discontinuation of an intravenous site. (323)

_____ 7. The patient's family may be permitted to bring in food for the patient if the facility is unable to provide the food. (Box 21.4)

_____ 8. A low-fat diet requires the elimination of all fatty foods. (315)

_____ 9. The patient should be instructed to eat low-calorie foods first and eat the high-calorie foods if still hungry. (Box 21.6)

_____ 10. The skills of basic intravenous (IV) needle insertion, adjusting IV flow rate, administering IV medications and maintaining an IV site require the knowledge of a nurse. (*Delegation & Documentation* Box 21.3)

SHORT ANSWER

Directions: Using your own words, answer each question in the space provided.

11. Identify five purposes of intravenous (IV) therapy. (320)

    a. _____

    b. _____

    c. _____

    d. _____

    e. _____

12. Identify three potential complications of IV therapy. (322)

    a. _____

    b. _____

    c. _____

13. Describe the causes of dehydration in older adults. (Box 21.2)

_____

_____

_____

_____

_____

_____

_____

_____

MULTIPLE CHOICE

Directions: Select the best answer(s) for each of the following questions.

14. A patient requires an increase in proteins in the diet. The patient care technician expects the nurse will recommend that the patient increase her intake of: (*Select all that apply.*) (Box 21.6)
    1. chicken.
    2. cheese.
    3. vegetables.
    4. fruit.
    5. fish.

15. A patient in the hospital who is placed on a clear liquid diet may have: (313)
    1. orange juice.
    2. gelatin.
    3. sherbet.
    4. creamed soup.

16. The patient care technician is preparing to feed a patient. Which is inappropriate for feeding the patient? (317 and *Procedure 21.1*)
    1. Offering the patient the bedpan before the meal.
    2. Placing the patient in a recumbent position.
    3. Providing opportunity for hand hygiene before the meal.
    4. Talking with the patient during the meal.

17. The mother asks about giving strained fruits to her infant. The patient care technician knows that this food should be introduced at around age: (368)
    1. 2 months.
    2. 6 months.
    3. 8 months.
    4. 12 months.

18. What are the patient care technician's responsibilities in promoting nutrition for patients? (*Select all that apply.*) (310)
    1. Assisting patients to eat
    2. Designing diet plans for patients with chronic health problems
    3. Recording the patient's intake
    4. Observing the patient for signs of poor nutrition
    5. Communicating dietary concerns to the nurse
    6. Monitoring laboratory values that are related to nutritional intake

19. Which patient should not be offered low-fat milk? (310)
    1. 15-year-old female with type 1 diabetes
    2. 26-year-old female who is in the third trimester of pregnancy
    3. 68-year-old female who has a hip fracture related to osteoporosis
    4. 18-month-old female who is transitioning to cow's milk
20. The best food source for calcium is: (314)
    1. milk.
    2. meat.
    3. whole grains.
    4. green leafy vegetables.
21. The best way to determine the patient's fluid balance is to: (320)
    1. assess vital signs.
    2. weigh the patient daily.
    3. monitor IV fluid intake.
    4. check diagnostic test results.

This page intentionally left blank

22 Assisting with Urinary Elimination

WORD SCRAMBLE

Directions: Unscramble the words that are related to performing various skills and then match the word to the correct clue below. (324)

Scrambled Term	Unscrambled Term	Correct Clue
1. zationtecatheri		
2. pbnaed		
3. lridesau nurie		
4. ralinu		
5. blaredd igatnirn		
6. continencein		
7. factodeine		

Clues for words used in performing various skills

a. Introducing a rubber or plastic tube into the body

b. The act of eliminating feces

c. A device for collecting urine from patients

d. Inability to control bowel or bladder

e. Device for receiving feces or urine from either male or female patients confined to bed

f. Amount of urine left in the bladder after the patient voids

g. The process of voluntary control over voiding

FILL IN THE BLANK SENTENCES

Directions: Complete each sentence by filling in the blank with the correct word or phrase.

8. Urinary elimination is a natural process that clears the body of _____ and aids in maintaining _____. (324)

9. _____ are usually provided for documentation of normal voiding and stools. (325)

10. The absorbent material in incontinence products is located _____ so as to collect the urine and prevent leaking through to the person's clothes. (327)

11. _____ is helpful when urinary incontinence results from the patient's decreased perception of bladder fullness or impaired voluntary motor control. (327)

12. After surgery, the health care provider usually orders the catheter removed after _____. (336)

13. When inserting a urinary catheter into a female patient, the patient care technician knows that it should be inserted _____ inches. (*Procedure 22.3*)

TRUE OR FALSE

Directions: Write T for true or F for false in the blanks provided.

_____ 14. Inserting and monitoring the catheter and output can be delegated to the patient care technician. (324)

_____ 15. Patients should always be left alone when using a bedpan or urinal. (325)

_____ 16. The bedside commode is useful at night and for the patient who is not able to walk to the bathroom easily. (325–326)

_____ 17. Urinary incontinence can occur as a result of weak muscle sphincters. (327)

_____ 18. Urinary catheterization cannot be delegated to unlicensed assistive personnel. (*Delegation and Documentation* Box 22.1)

_____ 19. Kegel exercises may also be used as part of a bladder training regimen. (336)

MULTIPLE CHOICE

Directions: Select the best answer(s) for each of the following questions.

20. The patient care technician has the opportunity to perform urinary catheterization for a patient. What should the patient care technician do first? (*Procedure 22.3*)
    1. Perform hand hygiene and don gloves.
    2. Explain the procedure to the patient.
    3. Obtain the necessary equipment.
    4. Check the health care provider's order.

21. In caring for patients, which action demonstrates the patient care technician's understanding and use of Standard Precautions? (*Injury & Illness Prevention* Box 22.1)
    1. Always checks the patient's armband and asks patient to state name
    2. Assesses the patient's understanding and teaches accordingly
    3. Performs hand hygiene before and after every patient encounter
    4. Evaluates the patient's response to and tolerance of the procedure

22. The patient care technician must perform catheter care. Prior to starting the procedure, the patient care technician raises the bed and lowers one side rail. What is the best rationale for this action? (*Procedure 22.5*)
    1. Ensures patient safety and comfort
    2. Promotes good body mechanics
    3. Facilitates visualization of body
    4. Adheres to standard procedure

23. The patient care technician has inserted the urinary catheter into the patient and while the balloon is being inflated, the patient expresses discomfort. The patient care technician should: (*Procedure 22.3*)
    1. remove the catheter and begin the procedure again.
    2. pull back on the catheter to determine tension.
    3. draw fluid out of the balloon and move the catheter forward.
    4. continue to inflate the balloon since discomfort is expected.

24. The volume of urine present in the bladder can be determined with a: (326)
    1. bedpan.
    2. urinal.
    3. ultrasound.
    4. bladder scanner.

25. The nurse delegates the removal of an indwelling urinary catheter to a patient care technician. Which action requires correction? (*Injury & Illness Prevention* Box 22.1)
    1. Explaining the burning sensation with the first voiding
    2. Obtaining a final urine specimen from the drainage bag
    3. Deflating the balloon and pinching the catheter
    4. Using clean gloves and performing perineal care

26. Identify how the patient care technician achieves the following before, during, and after the performance of a procedure.

a. Identify the patient: _____

_____

b. Reduce the spread of microorganisms: _____

_____

c. Provide privacy: _____

_____

d. Ensure the patient's safety: _____

_____

This page intentionally left blank

23 Assisting with Bowel Elimination

FILL IN THE BLANK SENTENCES

Directions: Complete each sentence by filling in the blank with the correct word or phrase.

1. Every patient should have a bowel movement at least every _____. (339)
2. _____ position is customary for defecation. (339)
3. Even when an ostomy pouch is adhering well, it is best to change it at least every _____ days to allow for observation of the stoma and the skin around the stoma. (344)
4. For an older adult, a diet containing at least _____ of dietary fiber per day adds bulk, weight, and form to stool and improves defecation. (Box 23.1)
5. Patients who are constipated, or are having trouble moving their bowels, may be prescribed a _____ _____. (340)
6. The maximum amount of fluid that should be administered to an adult during a tap-water enema is _____ _____. (*Procedure 23.1*)

TRUE OR FALSE

Directions: Write T for true or F for false in the blanks provided.

_____ 7. The patient care technician should complete each patient's abdominal evaluation on hospital admission. (339)

_____ 8. Anxiety or stress can contribute to difficulty with defecation. (339)

_____ 9. Assisting with bowel elimination is an appropriate skill set for the patient care technician to possess. (340)

_____ 10. Avoid cold water and harsh soaps when washing the skin around the ostomy. (*Illness & Injury Prevention* Box 23.1)

_____ 11. Proper stoma appearance is moist and reddish-pink. (*Procedure 23.2*)

SHORT ANSWER

Directions: Using your own words, answer each question in the space provided.

12. Describe some of the healthy and dangerous habits people have to promote elimination. What can the health care provider do to promote elimination for the hospitalized patient? For the bedridden patient? (339)

_____

_____

_____

_____

13. Describe the causes of constipation in older adults. What strategies can help improve defecation in older adults? (Box 23.1)

_____

_____

_____

_____

Directions: Select the best answer(s) for each of the following questions.

14. The patient care technician is caring for a patient who is often constipated. The patient asks what influences the frequency of bowel movements. Which factor(s) influence normal bowel elimination? (*Select all that apply.*) (339)
    1. Age
    2. Obesity
    3. Fluid intake
    4. Nutrition
    5. Activity level

15. A patient who has been admitted has difficulty with bowel elimination. The patient care technician knows that care for this patient should promote a normal pattern of elimination. Which would be appropriate? (339)
    1. Provide laxatives.
    2. Establish a routine for defecation.
    3. Increase fiber in the patient's diet.
    4. Regularly check on the patient to monitor defecation habits.

16. The patient care technician is preparing to administer an enema. In what order should the patient care technician perform the following steps? Label the first step with 1 and the last step with 8. (*Procedure 23.1*)
    _____ Perform hand hygiene and don PPE per CDC, OSHA, and facility guidelines.
    _____ Introduce yourself to the patient.
    _____ Close the door or pull privacy curtain.
    _____ Explain the procedure and the reason it is being done.
    _____ Check the health care provider's order.
    _____ Evaluate the patient.
    _____ Confirm the patient's identity.
    _____ Assemble equipment.

17. Ostomy pouches must be changed every 3–7 days to: (*Procedure 23.2*)
    1. prevent infection.
    2. prevent excess drainage.
    3. promote healing.
    4. prevent skin impairment.

18. Which statement is true regarding the management of hemorrhoids? (340)
    1. Avoid high-fiber foods.
    2. Avoid exercise or heavy activity.
    3. Use witch hazel pads for pain relief.
    4. Use laxatives to aid elimination.

24 Assisting with Oxygen Needs

FILL IN THE BLANK SENTENCES

Directions: Complete each sentence by filling in the blank with the correct word or phrase.

1. Oxygen is needed by _____ to metabolize nutrients and produce energy needed to function. (348)

2. For patients with a chronic lung disorder, flow rates higher than _____ L/min could eliminate the respiratory drive to breathe, and breathing may stop altogether. (Box 24.3)

3. Suctioning is performed as often as necessary, possibly every _____ during the first few postoperative hours. (*Injury and Illness Prevention* Box 24.2)

4. Have the patient practice coughing exercises 2–3 times every _____ while awake. (*Procedure 24.1*)

5. A(n) _____ is a simple, two-pronged device used to deliver low concentrations of oxygen. (*Procedure 24.4*)

TRUE OR FALSE

Directions: Write T for true or F for false in the blanks provided.

_____ 6. Brain damage resulting from the brain being deprived of oxygen can occur in minutes. (346)

_____ 7. Suctioning to keep the airway patent eliminates the need for the patient to perform coughing and deep-breathing exercises. (358)

_____ 8. The patient care technician is responsible for evaluating the patient's airway patency and informing the nurse. (*Delegation and Documentation* Box 24.2)

_____ 9. An incentive spirometer measures how deep a person can inhale and expand the lungs. (347)

_____ 10. Avoid the use of electrical appliances while oxygen is administered. (Box 24.1)

SHORT ANSWER

Directions: Using your own words, answer each question in the space provided.

11. Describe measures the patient care technician can take to reduce the older adult's risk for skin impairment when a nasal cannula is used for oxygen delivery. (Box 24.3)

12. Describe the positioning modification for patients with surgical incisions on the throat or abdomen. (*Procedure 24.1*)

Directions: Select the best answer(s) for each of the following questions.

13. The patient care technician knows that which patient could be at risk for airway interference? (346)
    1. An elderly patient
    2. A patient who just had surgery
    3. A patient who has difficulty chewing solids
    4. A patient who has a family history of sleep apnea

14. A patient receiving oxygen therapy has a nosebleed. The patient care technician knows that this is a result of: (348)
    1. hypoxia.
    2. an infection.
    3. high blood pressure.
    4. dry mucous membranes.

15. Preparation for tracheostomy care in the acute care environment includes: (*Procedure 24.3*)
    1. using clean technique and supplies for cleaning.
    2. preparing cotton balls to clean inside the ostomy.
    3. removing and cleaning the outer cannula.
    4. placing the patient in a semi-Fowler's position.

16. The patient care technician suspects hypoxia if the patient has which symptom(s)? (*Select all that apply.*) (Box 24.2)
    1. Pallor
    2. Restlessness
    3. Mood swings
    4. Decreased appetite
    5. Elevated blood pressure

17. The patient care technician is caring for a patient who is receiving oxygen therapy. The patient has elevated blood pressure and is restless. What should the patient care technician do? (349)
    1. Discontinue treatment.
    2. Note the ineffective breathing pattern.
    3. Document the observations.
    4. Notify the nurse immediately.

25 Blood Collecting and Processing

FILL IN THE BLANK SENTENCES

Directions: Fill in the blanks with the correct terms.

1. A blood draw ordered to be done immediately is a(n) _____ order. (363)
2. A laboratory paper used to collect a blood sample from newborns is a(n) _____. (379)
3. _____ is the liquid portion of whole blood that remains after the blood has clotted. (387)
4. _____ is the liquid portion of whole blood that contains active clotting agents. (363)
5. _____ is a situation in which the concentration of blood cells is increased in proportion to the plasma. (362)
6. _____ refers to fainting. (361)
7. _____ is the destruction or dissolution of red blood cells with a subsequent release of hemoglobin. (360)
8. _____ is a material that appears to be solid until subjected to a disturbance, such as centrifugation, at which point it becomes a liquid. (360)
9. _____ is when the blood is taken directly from a vein that is close to the surface of the skin. (361)

TABLE ACTIVITY

10. Complete the following table by providing actions that may make performing phlebotomy procedures on children less traumatic. (Table 25.7)

Age	Typical Mental State	Suggested Parental Involvement
Newborns (0–12 months)	Trust that adults will respond to their needs	
Infants and toddlers (1–3 years)	Minimal fear of danger but fear of separation; limited language and understanding of procedure	
Preschoolers (3–6 years)	Fearful of injury to body; still dependent on parent	
School-aged children (7–12 years)	Less dependent on parent and more willing to cooperate	
Teenagers (13–18 years)	Fully engaged in the process; embarrassed to show fear and may exhibit hostility to cover emotions	

MULTIPLE CHOICE

Directions: Select the best answer(s) for each of the following questions.

11. Which are causes of a hematoma? (*Select all that apply.*) (372)
    1. Allergic reaction
    2. Excessive probing to locate the vein
    3. Inserting the needle through the vein
    4. Infections or inflammations in the skin
    5. Failure to insert the needle far enough into the vein
12. In which circumstance(s) is a capillary puncture necessary? (*Select all that apply.*) (377)
    1. Young patients
    2. Underweight patients
    3. Patients who are dehydrated

4. Patients receiving intravenous therapy
5. Patients who require frequent glucose monitoring

13. The most commonly used antiseptic skin preparation for routine venipuncture is: (362)
    1. witch hazel.
    2. hydrogen peroxide.
    3. 70% isopropyl alcohol.
    4. povidone-iodine solution.

14. If a blood culture is ordered, additional preparation is needed at the venipuncture site to eliminate contaminating bacteria. What is commonly used for this skin preparation? (362)
    1. Hydrogen peroxide
    2. 70% isopropyl alcohol
    3. Povidone-iodine solution
    4. Chlorhexidine gluconate

15. Which strategy is appropriate for obtaining a blood draw from a patient with edema at the puncture site? (Table 25.4)
    1. Call for help.
    2. Loosen the tourniquet.
    3. Avoid the area; look for an alternate site.
    4. Adjust the depth of the needle and apply pressure.

16. Which are reasons the laboratory may reject a specimen? (*Select all that apply.*) (377)
    1. Defective tube
    2. Patient was anemic
    3. Insufficient quantity
    4. Improper handling
    5. Unlabeled or mislabeled specimen

17. The Clinical and Laboratory Standards Institute developed a set of standards outlining the order of blood draw for a multi-tube collection. Which tube would be filled first when blood is collected in a syringe? (364)
    1. Gray
    2. Yellow
    3. Light blue
    4. Lavender

18. For children younger than 1 year, dermal puncture is performed on the medial and lateral surfaces of the _____ of the heel. (379–380)
    1. top
    2. bottom
    3. left side
    4. right side

CASE STUDIES

19. One of Sophia's coworkers has just experienced a needle stick. What instruction should Sophia provide about care of the exposure site? (368)

_____

_____

_____

20. Noah is attending a conference on needle-stick prevention. List some of the ways accidental needle sticks can be prevented. (*Injury and Illness Prevention* Box 25.1)

_____

_____

_____

26 | Specimen Collecting and Testing

FILL IN THE BLANK SENTENCES

Directions: Fill in the blanks with the correct vocabulary terms from this chapter.

1. _____ Essential amino acid found in milk, eggs, and other foods. (397)
2. _____ Chemical reaction controlled by an enzyme. (398)
3. _____ White blood cells; leukocytes that have segmented nuclei; also known as *polymorphonuclear neutrophils* (PMNs) or *segmented neutrophils*. (399)
4. _____ White blood cells; leukocytes that have unsegmented nuclei; monocytes and lymphocytes in particular. (399)
5. _____ Level above which a substance cannot be reabsorbed by the renal tubules and therefore is excreted in the urine. (390)
6. _____ Fluid that remains after a liquid is passed through a membranous filter. (390)
7. _____ Strips used to test the specific gravity of urine. (397)
8. _____ Glucose test on a reagent strip. (400)
9. _____ Reagent tablets used to test for fat metabolism byproducts. (400)
10. _____ Substance detected in a positive pregnancy test. (400)
11. _____ Increases in the concentration of urine shortly before ovulation. (400–401)
12. _____ Procedure performed in the microbiology laboratory in which a specimen is cultured on artificial media to detect bacterial or fungal growth, followed by appropriate screening for antibiotic sensitivity. (402)
13. _____ Medical term for a urine sample with a persistent greenish-yellow foam that may indicate the patient has viral hepatitis. (396)
14. _____ Condition in which protein in the urine is in detectable amounts. (398)
15. _____ A common laboratory examination used to diagnose and treat disease that can reveal diseases of the bladder or kidney, systemic metabolic or endocrine disorders, and diseases of the liver or obstruction of the bile ducts. (390)
16. _____ The product of drug metabolism that is excreted into the urine. (401)

SHORT ANSWER

Directions: Using your own words, answer each question in the space provided.

17. Requesting a urine specimen may create an embarrassing moment for the patient. How can the patient care technician make this request without causing the patient undue discomfort? (390–391)

_____

_____

_____

18. List and describe six different methods of collecting a urine specimen. (391–392)

a. _____

_____

b. _____

_____

c. _____

_____

d. _____

_____

e. _____

_____

f. _____

_____

19. Define adulteration. How may urine be altered to affect the results of the drug test? What methods can detect alterations to the urine? (401–402)

_____

_____

_____

_____

_____

MULTIPLE CHOICE

Directions: Select the best answer(s) for each of the following questions.

20. What is the specific gravity of distilled water? (397)
    1. 1.000
    2. 1.005
    3. 1.010
    4. 1.025

21. Which statement is accurate about waived testing? (397)
    1. Must be simple
    2. Test must be error-proof
    3. Test must be available over the counter
    4. Cannot have potential for serious health impacts

22. A urine specimen with a pH below 7: (398)
    1. is neutral.
    2. indicates acidity.
    3. indicates alkalinity.
    4. indicates presence of bacteria.

23. The patient education instruction sheet should include the: (404)
    1. purpose of the test.
    2. side effects of the test.
    3. duration of the test.
    4. supplies needed for the test.

24. What does a nephron include? (Figure 26.1)
    1. Bladder
    2. Ureter
    3. Kidney
    4. Glomerulus

25. A patient brings a urine sample to the office in an old "pill bottle." Should Rosa, the patient care technician, accept the urine sample for testing? Why or why not? What patient education guidelines for collecting a urine sample at home should Rosa provide this patient? (Box 26.1)

   _____

   _____

   _____

   _____

   _____

26. Dan is responsible for orienting a new employee to drug testing and chain of custody procedures in Dr. Hill's office. Summarize these guidelines. (*Delegation and Documentation* Box 26.1)

   _____

   _____

   _____

   _____

   _____

   _____

   _____

27 Care for the Surgical Patient

TRUE OR FALSE

Directions: Write T for true or F for false in the blanks provided.

1. _____ Air currents carry bacteria, so body motions over a sterile field and talking should be kept to a minimum. (414)
2. _____ Infection can cause death in some circumstances. (413)
3. _____ A sterile field can get wet but remain microorganism-free. (Rules for Maintaining a Sterile Field box on page 414)
4. _____ Sterile team members should always face each other. (Rules for Maintaining a Sterile Field box on page 414)
5. _____ You should always keep the sterile field in your view. (Rules for Maintaining a Sterile Field box on page 414)
6. _____ You should never turn your back on a sterile field or wander away from it. (Rules for Maintaining a Sterile Field box on page 414)
7. _____ Autoclave tape contains a chemical dye that changes color when exposed to steam. (410)
8. _____ Nonsterile individuals should never reach over a sterile field. (Rules for Maintaining a Sterile Field box on page 414)
9. _____ Storage practices for sterilized instruments must be date-related. (410)
10. _____ The recommended temperature for sterilization in an autoclave is 121–123 °C (250–255 °F). (409)

SHORT ANSWER

Directions: Using your own words, answer each question in the space provided.

11. Explain the difference between surgical and medical asepsis. When is each performed? (418)

_____

_____

_____

_____

12. What guidelines should be followed when the autoclave is unloaded? (410)

_____

_____

_____

_____

13. Melissa is preparing a patient for a procedure and the patient seems anxious and worried. What can Melissa do to support the patient? (411–412)

_____

_____

_____

_____

14. Describe the importance of skin preparation and describe how it is done. (*Procedure 27.1*)

_____

_____

_____

_____

MULTIPLE CHOICE

Directions: Select the best answer(s) for each of the following questions.

15. _____ refers to destruction of pathogens by physical or chemical means. (418)
    1. Hand hygiene
    2. Disinfection
    3. Sanitization
    4. Sterilization

16. Personal protective equipment for autoclave procedures includes: (*Select all that apply.*) (409)
    1. fluid-resistant gloves.
    2. a face shield and/or goggles.
    3. heat-resistant boots or shoes.
    4. heat-resistant autoclave gloves.
    5. a laboratory coat or impervious gown.

17. The main cause of incomplete sterilization in an autoclave is the presence of _____. (410)
    1. steam
    2. bacteria
    3. residual air
    4. air that is too warm

18. What is the shelf life of polypropylene autoclave bags? (411)
    1. 28 days
    2. 30 days
    3. 3 months
    4. 6 months

19. Which surgical procedure uses a high-frequency current to cut through tissue and coagulate blood vessels? (411)
    1. Laser
    2. Microsurgery
    3. Electrosurgery
    4. Endoscopic

20. The human skin is a reservoir of _____, but it cannot be sterilized without the risk of damaging cells and tissues. (412)
    1. germs
    2. viruses
    3. Staph
    4. bacteria

21. Which is a reason for applying a sterile dressing? (415)
    1. Expedite wound healing
    2. Prevent bleeding and swelling
    3. Hold the wound edges together
    4. Protect area surrounding the wound

22. Which surgical procedure uses a fiberoptic instrument with a miniature camera mounted on a flexible tube to examine the inside of an organ or cavity? (418)
    1. Cryosurgery
    2. Microsurgery
    3. Electrosurgery
    4. Endoscopic

28 Heat and Cold Applications

TRUE OR FALSE

Directions: Write T for true or F for false in the blanks provided.

1. _____ The application of heat or cold affects the blood circulating throughout the body. (419)
2. _____ The patient care technician can determine when it is appropriate to use heat and/or cold therapy. (419)
3. _____ The physician's order for heat therapy should include frequency and specify a temperature. (420)
4. _____ Tissue damage resulting from cold is often accompanied by a burning type of pain. (420)
5. _____ Moist heat is a better conductor of heat than dry heat. (420)

FILL IN THE BLANK SENTENCES

Directions: Complete each sentence by filling in the blank with the correct word or phrase.

6. The body's reaction to heat therapy can include a rapid pulse, _____, or difficulty breathing. (420)
7. Typically, patients exposed to temperatures above _____ experience pain and burning. (419)
8. _____ applications are generally used to provide comfort and speed healing. (419)
9. Heat applications left in place for more than _____ can cause vessels to constrict, which decreases blood flow to that area. (420)
10. Contraindications to heat therapy include any bleeding, _____, and cardiovascular problems. (420)

SHORT ANSWER

Directions: Using your own words, answer the question in the space provided.

11. Identify patients at greatest risk for developing injuries related to heat and cold applications. What measures should the patient care technician take to prevent injury to patients with heat and cold applications? (*Injury & Illness Prevention* Box 28.1 *and Delegation and Documentation* Box 28.1)

   _____

   _____

   _____

   _____

Directions: Select the best answer(s) for each of the following questions.

12. The patient was diagnosed with a sprained ankle and the health care provider recommended a cold application for 20 minutes. Which condition would cause the patient care technician to question the order? (420)
    1. The patient's ankle is already slightly swollen.
    2. The pain medication has not had time to work.
    3. The patient has a history of peripheral vascular disease.
    4. The patient tells the patient care technician that 20 minutes is too long.

13. A cold application is ordered for the patient. The patient care technician is aware that a positive effect of this treatment is: (423)
    1. vasodilation.
    2. local anesthesia.
    3. reduced blood viscosity.
    4. increased metabolism.

14. The patient care technician applies heat to a fairly large area on the patient's trunk. The patient reports feeling slightly dizzy and his pulse is rapid. What is the best physiologic explanation for this systemic reaction? (419)
    1. The heat application has triggered a fever.
    2. The trunk contains some large blood vessels.
    3. The application is causing vasodilation.
    4. Antibodies and leukocytes are activated.

15. The patient care technician is observing a family member assist the patient with a heat pad. The patient care technician would intervene if the family member performs which action? (422)
    1. Assists the patient to lie on the heating pad
    2. Adjusts the pad to the lowest temperature setting
    3. Places a cloth between the skin and the heating device
    4. Checks electrical cord for fraying or kinks

16. The health care provider has ordered the application of a warm compress to a patient's leg wound. What does the patient care technician tell the patient about the compress? (423)
    1. "We soak your leg in a warm solution that has antibiotic medication for at least 30 minutes a day."
    2. "We wrap your leg with a towel and then apply a dry heating device that is similar to a heating pad."
    3. "We apply a hot water bottle to your leg and then wrap a towel around it to retain the warmth."
    4. "We apply a sterile, moist gauze dressing to the wound, then wrap it with a warm waterproof heating pad."

Student Name_____ Date_____

29 Care of Wounds and Pressure Ulcers

MATCHING

Directions: Match the term on the left with the descriptions on the right. Indicate your answers in the spaces provided. (425)

Term	Description
_____ 1. dehiscence	a. A bandage that is made of large pieces of material to fit a specific body part
_____ 2. T-tube	b. The formation of new cells during wound healing
_____ 3. binder	c. A drainage tube into the duct to maintain free flow of bile
_____ 4. purulent	d. The softening and breaking down of skin resulting from prolonged exposure to moisture
_____ 5. epithelialization	e. Removal of fluids from a body cavity, wound or other source of discharge by one or more methods.
_____ 6. macerated	f. Rupture of the wound at the incisional line
_____ 7. Sanguineous	g. Bright-red wound drainage
_____ 8. drainage	h. Producing or containing pus

SHORT ANSWER

Directions: Using your own words, answer each question in the space provided.

9. What are the time frames and characteristics of the three phases of wound healing? (426)

   a. Inflammatory phase: _____

   b. Reconstruction phase: _____

   c. Maturation phase: _____

10. Describe the three types of wound healing. (426)

    a. Primary: _____

    b. Secondary: _____

    c. Tertiary: _____

11. What is the purpose of each of the following types of dressings? (430)

    a. Gauze: _____

    b. Semiocclusive: _____

    c. Occlusive: _____

    d. Dry dressing: _____

    e. Transparent: _____

12. Identify factors that may impair wound healing. (425) _____

_____

_____

_____

_____

Directions: Select the best answer(s) for each of the following questions.

13. Which lunch tray is best for providing protein, vitamins A and C, and zinc, the nutrients required for wound healing? (426)
    1. A peanut butter sandwich with a glass of milk
    2. A bowl of bean soup with crackers and iced tea
    3. Broiled seafood with spinach salad and tomato juice
    4. Stir-fried mixed vegetables with rice and hot tea

14. The patient has no contraindications for fluid intake; over a 24-hour period, he drank 16 ounces of decaffeinated coffee, 10 ounces of juice, 6 ounces of milk, and a half a liter of soda. What instructions does the patient care technician give the patient about fluid intake to promote wound healing? (427)
    1. Instructs the patient to continue drinking the same amount as he drank today
    2. Tells the patient that tomorrow he should try to drink twice as much as today
    3. Advises the patient that drinking excessive fluid is likely to decrease appetite for food
    4. Suggests that he drinks 2–3 additional 8-oz servings of his favorite fluid every day

15. The patient care technician is caring for a patient who has a large abdominal incision. The patient tells the patient care technician that she is afraid to sit up or even move because of the pain and the strain on the incision site. What instructions should the patient care technician give to the patient? (427)
    1. "Rest in bed until the incision site is less tender and healing has progressed."
    2. "Roll to one side, use your elbow as a lever, and push to a sitting position."
    3. "Hold a pillow next to your abdomen and roll forward into a sitting position."
    4. "Call for assistance whenever needed and someone will help you sit up."

16. A patient has just returned from surgery. After the first 4 hours, the patient care technician expects the nurse will inspect the dressings every _____ hours during the first 24 hours. (427)
    1. 1 to 2   2. 1 to 3   3. 2 to 3   4. 2 to 4

17. Which patient is most likely to benefit from the application of a triangular binder? (*Procedure 28.2*)
    1. Has a chronic pressure ulcer on the sacral area
    2. Has a possible fracture of the forearm
    3. Has venous stasis ulcer on left ankle
    4. Has a surgical wound on the lateral chest area

18. The patient care technician is preparing to change the patient's dry sterile dressing. Upon attempting to remove the old dressing, it adheres to the site. What should the patient care technician do? (430)
    1. Notify the health care provider.   3. Pull the dressing off quickly.
    2. Leave the dressing in place.   4. Moisten the dressing with saline.

19. The patient returned to the unit 3 hours ago after having surgery on the abdomen, and the dressing is now saturated with red, watery drainage. What should the patient care technician do first? (428)
    1. Notify the nurse and the health care provider.
    2. Take the patient's vital signs and assess for pain.
    3. Securely reinforce the dressing with layers of gauze.
    4. Remove the dressing and observe the wound site.

20. From 9:00 AM until now, 11:40 PM, 650 mL has drained from a patient's surgical wound. What should the patient care technician do first? (428)
    1. Record the amount and appearance of the drainage and continue to observe.
    2. Take the patient's vital signs, assess for other symptoms, and inform the provider.
    3. Make sure that the patient's linens are clean and dry and empty the drainage receptacle.
    4. Apply a pressure dressing and place the patient in a supine position.

21. The patient needs an abdominal binder. What is the most important consideration when implementing this application? (431)
    1. Respiratory function must not be restricted.
    2. Vomiting and nausea are a contraindication.
    3. Binders cannot be used for patients who are obese.
    4. Older patients have difficulty tolerating the binder.

22. The patient care technician is applying a dressing over the insertion site of a peripheral intravenous catheter. Which dressing is the best choice? (431)
    1. Sterile tape with dry gauze
    2. Moistened gauze with paper tape
    3. Transparent dressing
    4. Sterile pad with chevron taping

30 Rehabilitative and Restorative Care

MATCHING

Directions: Match the terms on the left to the correct definition on the right. (438)

Term	Definition
_____ 1. impairment	a. Any restriction in or lack of ability to perform an activity in the manner or within the range considered normal as the result of impairment
_____ 2. disability	b. Irreversible lifelong disease state or impairment
_____ 3. handicap	c. Loss or abnormality of psychological, physical, or anatomic structure or function
_____ 4. functional limitation	d. Physical, mental, or emotional impairment or disability that interferes with one's normal functioning
_____ 5. chronic illness	e. Loss of ability to perform tasks or activities of daily living

FILL IN THE BLANK SENTENCES

Directions: Complete each sentence by filling in the blank with the correct word or phrase.

6. Emphasis on acute care persists, despite the fact that people with _____ constitute the largest group of health consumers. (439)

7. Rehabilitation services for the older person are built around maintaining _____ abilities, ensuring safety, promoting effective coping, preventing _____, and modifying the _____ for maximum independence. (440)

8. A disability has a number of potential effects on both the patient and the family, including _____ and emotional changes and changes in roles, body _____, self-concept, and family _____. (440)

9. Rehabilitation is a(n) _____ process. (440)

10. Individuals with disabilities do not always accept their disability; learning to _____ to the circumstances is a positive method of coping. (440)

11. The role of a rehabilitation nurse is to put the individual in _____ of his or her own care rather than taking charge. (442)

12. It is important to recognize that having a disability is just one of many _____ of the normal human experience. (445)

13. The primary difference between rehabilitation of children and rehabilitation of adults is the _____ of the child. (447)

14. Studies of resource allocation show that _____ rehabilitation saves thousands of dollars and increases the chance of the individual being able to live independently. (443)

MULTIPLE CHOICE

Directions: Select the best answer(s) for each of the following questions.

15. The patient experienced a spinal cord injury at the T1–T5 level. The patient care technician anticipates that the patient should be able to: (445)
    1. assist with activities of daily living (ADLs).
    2. ambulate with the use of assistive devices.
    3. resume normal sexual activities.
    4. control bowel and bladder function.

91

16. The construction worker sustained an injury to C3 after a fall at a work site. The patient care technician anticipates that this patient will have: (445)
    1. use of the arms, but not the legs.
    2. control of bladder, but not bowels.
    3. potential for respiratory failure and infections.
    4. problems understanding and following instructions.

17. The spouse reports that the patient tripped and bumped his head. He never lost consciousness, but seemed confused for a few minutes after the accident. Which assessment finding does the patient care technician expect the nurse to find? (446)
    1. Headache and vertigo
    2. Difficulty with judgment and reasoning
    3. Posttrauma amnesia and aggressiveness
    4. Appears awake, but does not respond

18. The patient care technician is assisting a nurse in assessing a patient who had a stroke and was recently admitted to the rehabilitation unit. The patient care technician knows that the best method to determine how much assistance is required for hygienic care is: (442)
    1. ask the unlicensed assistive personnel (UAP) to go with the patient and assist as needed.
    2. ask the patient how much he feels like he can do for himself.
    3. read the documentation from the transferring facility.
    4. observe the patient as he performs tasks such as eating.

19. The elderly patient with a hip fracture has challenges related to bathing due to problems with ambulation and balance. Which action would foster independence and ensure safety? (442)
    1. Help the patient sit in the bathtub and bathe self, rather than attempt to stand and balance in the shower.
    2. Have the UAP stay with the patient for the whole time it takes for showering, but tell the UAP to let the patient wash herself.
    3. Have the patient remain in bed and bring her a basin of water and towels and allow her to wash her own hands and face.
    4. Assist the patient to sit in a stable chair in the shower stall and adjust the water temperature of the handheld shower spray.

20. Which patient is most likely to need minimization of distractions that would prevent participation in therapy? (445)
    1. Patient who has been depressed for several months
    2. Patient who had a myocardial infarction
    3. Patient who had a traumatic brain injury
    4. Patient who has chronic obstructive pulmonary disease

21. A patient was involved in an explosion at a chemical factory and sustained polytrauma/blast-related injury (PT/BRI). What type(s) of injuries would the health care team expect to find? (*Select all that apply.*) (444)
    1. Burns
    2. Fractures of extremities
    3. Amputations
    4. Brain injury
    5. Myocardial infarction
    6. Hearing loss

CRITICAL THINKING ACTIVITY

22. The patient care technician is assisting the nurse in caring for a patient who sustained a traumatic brain injury in a motor vehicle accident. The patient was admitted to an acute care facility immediately after the accident. Now that the patient is stable, he has been transferred to a rehabilitation facility. The patient is alert and ambulatory, but suffers residual effects from the brain injury.
    a. In the rehabilitative assessment of this patient, what may the patient care technician expect the nurse to find? (447)

    _____

    _____

    _____

    _____

b. What type of interventions does the patient care technician anticipate for the patient with a traumatic brain injury? (447)

_____

_____

_____

_____

_____

_____

This page intentionally left blank

31 Care of Women and Children

FILL IN THE BLANK SENTENCES

Directions: Complete each sentence by filling in the blank with the correct word or phrase.

1. The _____ lasts about 3–6 weeks, from the time the woman delivers the placenta until the reproductive organs return to the nonpregnant size and position. (454)

2. The _____ is an upside-down, pear-shaped muscular organ, and its sole purpose is to house and nourish the fetus from implantation shortly after conception until parturition. (451)

3. The tissue of light-skinned women, especially those with reddish hair, is not as readily _____ _____ as that of darker-skinned women, and healing may be less efficient. (456)

4. The newborn's head is disproportionately _____ for the body. (459)

5. The newborn's hematocrit may range from _____. (459)

6. Playing pretend and making a game out of an examination visit is the appropriate technique for a(n) _____ _____ child. (465)

7. The younger the child, the _____ the pulse. (465)

8. Healed lacerations from childbirth are common in a(n) _____ patient. (454)

9. Expectant mothers begin to leak _____ in the later weeks of the third trimester. (456)

10. _____ is the thinning of the cervix from its prelabor length of 1 to 1½ inches to a completely thin tissue. (454)

TABLE ACTIVITY

11. Directions: Complete the table below with the expected values for the newborn. (459)

Assessment of Newborn	Normal Value
Head circumference	
Relationship of head to chest circumference	
Temperature	
Pulse	
Respirations	
Blood pressure	

SHORT ANSWER

Directions: Using your own words, answer the question in the space provided.

12. Describe the signs of child abuse. What should the patient care technician do if he or she suspects child abuse? (468, Box 31.5)

_____

_____

_____

_____

Directions: Select the best answer(s) for each of the following questions.

13. Care of the circumcision includes: (462)
    1. removing the yellow crusting right away.
    2. applying the diaper loosely.
    3. assessing for bleeding every hour for 4 hours.
    4. using petroleum gauze under the Plastibell.

14. An appropriate technique to teach the new mother about the baby's bath is: (461)
    1. vigorous removal of the vernix caseosa.
    2. use of plain water on the perineal area.
    3. washing the baby twice daily.
    4. having the bathwater at 100 °F (37.7 °C).

15. What information should be provided to the mother regarding sexuality? (454–456)
    1. Menses usually return in 3–5 months.
    2. Breastfeeding acts as an effective contraceptive.
    3. Discomfort and bleeding are expected with sexual activity.
    4. Avoid sexual activity until after the first postpartum office visit.

16. What color drainage might a woman expect to find up to 6 days after delivery? (456)
    1. Bright-red blood with tissue
    2. Thin pinkish-brown drainage
    3. Slightly yellow to white drainage
    4. Small clots with a fleshy odor

17. The postpartum patient complains of a persistent headache. Which action should be performed first? (458)
    1. Obtain an order for a mild analgesic, such as acetaminophen.
    2. Reassure that pregnancy-induced headaches will abate.
    3. Check the blood pressure and compare it to baseline measurements.
    4. Check the record for history of epidural or spinal anesthesia.

18. A patient who had a cesarean section received liquids for the first day with a gradual reintroduction to a regular diet. The patient care technician knows that the nurse would do what to determine whether to offer the patient solid foods? (457)
    1. Follow the protocol or clinical pathway for cesarean section patients.
    2. Give solid food when the dietary kitchen includes it on the meal tray.
    3. Call the health care provider and clarify specific parameters.
    4. Assess the abdomen and auscultate for bowel sounds.

19. The patient received an epidural block. In the early recovery stage, what would be considered a normal finding? (458)
    1. Decreased sensation in both legs
    2. Altered level of consciousness
    3. Elevated blood pressure compared to baseline
    4. Low-grade fever

20. The woman's temperature is slightly elevated 12 hours after delivery of the baby. What additional assessment does the patient care technician anticipate that the nurse will perform first? (458)
    1. Check the appearance and odor of the lochia.
    2. Assess skin turgor and condition of mucous membranes.
    3. Palpate the fundus for height and firmness.
    4. Check a urine specimen for foul odor and cloudiness.

21. The patient care technician tells the nurse that there was a gush of brownish vaginal drainage when the patient got out of bed and stood up. What will the nurse likely do first? (453)
    1. Inform the patient care technician that secretions pool in the supine position and flow is expected.
    2. Ask the patient care technician to describe the amount and color of the drainage and the patient's response.
    3. Check on the patient and assess for pain, dizziness, or continued vaginal flow.
    4. Tell the patient that there is nothing to worry about and help her clean up.

32 Caring for the Older Adult

MATCHING

Directions: Match the following terms with their definitions.

Definitions	Terms
_____ 1. The secretion or discharge of tears	a. collagen (471)
_____ 2. The severe loss of intellectual ability	b. Alzheimer's disease (476)
_____ 3. A difficulty in being able to focus on detailed objects close at hand	c. dementia (475)
_____ 4. Protein that forms the inelastic fibers of tendons, ligaments, and fascia	d. elastin (471)
_____ 5. A progressive deterioration of the brain caused by the destruction of central nervous system neurons	e. lacrimation (471)
_____ 6. A decreased ability to hear high frequencies and to discriminate sounds; age-related hearing loss	f. seborrheic keratoses (474)
_____ 7. An essential part of elastic connective tissue that is flexible and elastic when moist	g. presbyopia (471)
_____ 8. Waxy, greasy papules on the skin that vary from tan to dark brown; also called *age spots*	h. presbycusis (471)

SHORT ANSWER

Directions: Using your own words, answer each question in the space provided.

9. The patient, Mary, is concerned about her risk for osteoporosis. What can Bill, the patient care technician, tell Mary about common risk factors for the development of osteoporosis? Can she do anything to prevent the decrease in bone density? What tests are done to diagnose osteoporosis? Describe methods for preventing and treating osteoporosis. (474)

_____

_____

_____

10. List six suggestions for helping elderly individuals prevent and treat dry skin. (474)

a. _____

b. _____

c. _____

d. _____

e. _____

f. _____

11. List six suggestions for helping an older adult with mobility, dexterity, and balance. (Box 32.3)

a. _____

b. _____

c. _____

d. _____

e. _____

f. _____

12. Summarize the patient care technician's role in caring for elderly patients. (480–481) _____

_____

_____

_____

13. Explain four age-related changes that occur in the anatomic structures of the eye. (Table 32.2)

_____

_____

_____

14. Describe the geriatric depression scale. Why is it a helpful tool for assessing the mental health of aging people? (478–479)

_____

_____

_____

MULTIPLE CHOICE

Directions: Select the best answer(s) for each of the following questions.

15. The 5-minute test designed to evaluate basic mental function in a number of different areas is known as the: (476)
    1. Cognitive Function Test.
    2. Mini-Mental State Examination.
    3. Geriatric Mental Function Test.
    4. Mini-Mental Geriatric Examination.

16. Which statement(s) is/are accurate about aging? (*Select all that apply.*) (Box 32.1)
    1. Most aging people will develop dementia.
    2. Aging people are more likely to have health issues.
    3. Older workers are less productive than younger ones.
    4. Sexual interest declines significantly with age.
    5. At any given time, approximately 5% of the aging population lives in long-term facilities.

17. The patient care technician is talking to the daughter of a woman who has Alzheimer's disease. The daughter says that her mother is able to care for herself but often repeats statements, has difficulty reading and writing, and has become increasingly paranoid and cranky. What stage of Alzheimer's is the mother exhibiting? (Box 32.5)
    1. First stage
    2. Second stage
    3. Third stage
    4. Fourth stage

18. Which is an accurate description of a change that occurs in the pulmonary system with aging? (476)
    1. Increased coughing
    2. Expanded area for gas exchange in the lungs
    3. Steady vital capacity
    4. Weakened respiratory muscles

19. Which is an accurate description of a change that occurs in the cardiovascular system with aging? (472)
    1. Decreased blood pressure
    2. Myocardial cells reduce in size
    3. Difficulty clearing mucus from the lungs
    4. Vessel walls thicken and become less elastic

33 Caring for Patients with Mental Health Needs

FILL IN THE BLANK SENTENCES

Directions: Complete each sentence by filling in the blank with the correct word or phrase.

1. _____ often consists of a pattern of behaviors that are obvious, threatening, and disruptive to relationships or are very different from behaviors considered socially and culturally acceptable. (486)

2. An astounding _____ of people in the U.S. will develop a mental health disorder in their lifetime. (486)

3. Maladaptive behavior is often part of a response to acute _____. (487)

4. _____ often serves as a gateway drug. (490)

5. The removal of the poisonous effects of a substance is called _____. (491)

6. The fastest growing section of the homeless population is the _____. (492)

MULTIPLE CHOICE

Directions: Select the best answer(s) for each of the following questions.

7. A parent had a bad day at work and comes home and shouts at the children. This is an example of which defense mechanism? (485)
   1. Projection
   2. Displacement
   3. Identification
   4. Reaction formation

8. Which person is demonstrating regression? (486)
   1. Victim of sexual abuse laughs while telling about the incident.
   2. Aggressive adolescent participates in a lot of competitive sports.
   3. An 80-year-old acts as if an incident of incontinence did not occur.
   4. An 8-year-old sucks his thumb when hospitalized for the first time.

9. An adolescent female patient tells the patient care technician that she often feels very "uneasy," but can't identify any specific reasons for this feeling. This patient is experiencing: (487)
   1. stress.
   2. anxiety.
   3. crisis.
   4. mental illness.

10. Based on factors that possibly affect mental health, which adolescent is most likely to have the best mental health later in life? (486)
    1. Participates in several school activities and has reasonably good grades
    2. Very competitive in sports and especially eager to be better than older brother
    3. Has a successful father, but mother died shortly after adolescent was born
    4. Has exceptional academic record and parents expect superior performance in all areas

11. Which statement made at a substance abuse support group is evidence of the best level of mental health? (491)
    1. "I don't have any problems with drinking anymore."
    2. "I just try to avoid drinking, one day at a time."
    3. "As long as my wife doesn't drink, then I won't drink either."
    4. "I've had a really hard time in life and I don't like being judged."

12. What is the best rationale for all patient care technicians to study and be familiar with the concepts of basic mental health? (486)
    1. Every patient care technician must study mental health concepts to pass the licensure examination.
    2. Patient care technicians need excellent mental health in order to help their patients.
    3. Patient care technicians have daily contact with patients who are at risk for mental health problems.
    4. Younger patient care technicians may lack personal experience in dealing with loss or mental illness.

13. There is a fire in the facility and the patient care technician is attempting to instruct patients to go to a safe area. Which patient is least likely to be able to understand and appropriately respond to a simple command? (Box 33.2)
    1. Using a wheelchair to assist bedbound roommate to safe area
    2. Frantically searching through belongings to find her wedding ring
    3. Standing in the corner, crying and clinging to the bedrail
    4. Walking towards safe area, but arguing about the need to leave

14. Which student is most likely to experience stress during the final examination for a course? (487)
    1. Has done well throughout the semester, but didn't get much sleep the night before the exam
    2. Knows that the test is important, but believes that test is just another hurdle to get over
    3. Is smart and a good student, has children, works full-time, and spouse has chronic illness
    4. Has studied hard for final examination, but graduating is contingent on test results

15. A newly admitted patient appears upset. She says, "I'm going to wear my own clothes. I'm not going to answer any more questions and I'm not giving anyone any blood or pee or anything else!" How should the patient care technician respond? (491)
    1. "You can wear your own nightgown if you would prefer."
    2. "Let me call your health care provider, so you can talk to him."
    3. "Coming into the hospital is really difficult. What can I do to help?"
    4. "Looks like you are having a bad time. I'll come back later."

16. The son of an elderly woman who lives in a long-term care facility reports that his mother seems to get sick whenever he tries to take vacation time with his wife. He feels frustrated, but also guilty, so he doesn't leave. What should the patient care technician do first? (491)
    1. Validate the son's feelings of frustration and guilt and offer emotional support.
    2. Reassure the elderly mother that she will be well cared for while her son is gone.
    3. Suggest that the son take an overnight trip as a trial run for everyone.
    4. Tell the son that the mother is manifesting a secondary gain by being sick.

CRITICAL THINKING ACTIVITY

17. Think about times in the past where you have witnessed (or personally experienced) various levels of anxiety. Briefly describe the behaviors that you observed (or feelings that you personally experienced) in each case. (Box 33.2)

    a. Mild anxiety: _____

    _____

    b. Moderate anxiety: _____

    _____

    c. Severe anxiety: _____

    _____

    d. Panic: _____

    _____

    e. Refer back to the situation of mild anxiety that you just described. What coping responses were used by the individual to deal with stress? (487)

    _____

    _____

    _____

    f. What would you do to strengthen the healthy coping mechanisms and alter or adapt the unhealthy or overused coping mechanism for that person? (487)

    _____

    _____

    _____

34 Caring for Patients with Chronic Conditions

FILL IN THE BLANK SENTENCES

Directions: Complete each sentence by filling in the blank with the correct word or phrase.

1. A(n) _____ occurs when a vessel in the brain either ruptures or becomes blocked and the tissue served by the damaged vessel is deprived of oxygen. (494)

2. _____ cancer is the leading cause of cancer-related deaths for both men and women in the United States. (501)

3. A positive _____ reaction indicates the possibility of active or latent tuberculosis or exposure to the disease. (497)

4. Chronic tissue hypoxia can lead to an abnormal enlargement of the ends of the fingers called _____. (Figure 34.3)

5. Atherosclerotic plaque buildup is primarily related to _____ blood levels. (501)

SHORT ANSWER

Directions: Using your own words, answer each question in the space provided.

6. Define the four tests used to diagnose **tuberculosis**. (496)

    a. _____

    b. _____

    c. _____

    d. _____

7. Discuss the difference between latent and active tuberculosis. (Box 34.2)_____

    _____

    _____

    _____

    _____

8. Discuss how tuberculosis is treated. (496–497)_____

    _____

    _____

    _____

    _____

9. Explain what happens during an asthma attack and how the patient should be treated. (498)

    _____

    _____

    _____

101

10. You are responsible for teaching a patient how to use an inhaler. Explain the procedure. (Box 34.3)

_____

_____

_____

_____

MULTIPLE CHOICE

Directions: Select the best answer(s) for each of the following questions.

11. Carcinoma of the _____ is pathologically linked to smoking and chronic alcohol consumption. (501)
    1. lung
    2. larynx
    3. pharynx
    4. paranasal sinuses

12. Tissue inflammation caused by asthma would be treated with: (498)
    1. alteplase.
    2. albuterol.
    3. fluticasone.
    4. ipratropium bromide.

13. Which are signs and symptoms of obstructive sleep apnea? (*Select all that apply.*) (500)
    1. Narcolepsy
    2. Congestion
    3. Hypersomnia
    4. Morning headache
    5. Dry mouth on awakening

14. Recurrent inflammation of the membranes lining the bronchial tubes describes: (497)
    1. asthma.
    2. emphysema.
    3. tuberculosis.
    4. chronic bronchitis.

15. Signs and symptoms of a heart attack in women include: (*Select all that apply.*) (Box 34.6)
    1. nausea.
    2. jaw pain.
    3. dizziness.
    4. headache.
    5. shortness of breath.

35 End-of-Life Care

FILL IN THE BLANK SENTENCES

Directions: Complete each sentence by filling in the blank with the correct word or phrase.

1. _____ is a period of mourning or an expression of grief in reaction to the death of some-one close. (514)

2. _____ is aggressive care in which the goal is curing the disease and prolonging life at all costs. (511)

3. The Hospice Medicare Benefit covers all expenses for palliative care related to terminal illness, including _____, _____, _____, _____, and _____ care. (Box 35.2)

4. _____ is appropriate when a cure is not possible, but care is still necessary. (521)

5. It is possible to begin palliative care earlier in the dying process, whereas hospice is usually available only _____ of life. (510)

TABLE ACTIVITY

6. Directions: Complete the table below with the functions or responsibilities of the Core Interdisciplinary Hospice Team. (Table 35.1)

Core Interdisciplinary Hospice Team	
Team Member	Function or Responsibility
a. Medical director	
b. Nurse coordinator	
c. Social worker	
d. Spiritual coordinator	

MULTIPLE CHOICE

Directions: Select the best answer(s) for each of the following questions.

7. Signs and symptoms expected in the patient nearing death include: (*Select all that apply.*) (Table 35.3)
   1. lowered blood pressure.
   2. rapid, bounding pulse.
   3. irregular respiratory pattern.
   4. mouth-breathing with dry mucous membranes.
   5. rapid, anxious eye movements.

8. The patient tells the patient care technician that he has some "papers" with his end-of-life preferences. To what document is the patient referring? (520)
   1. A will
   2. Advance directive
   3. Health care contract
   4. Designation of durable power of attorney

9. Number the following actions in the order they should be done for postmortem care, from first to last. (*Procedure 35.1*)

_____ a. Remove or secure all tubings according to policy.

_____ b. Wash hands and don gloves.

_____ c. Place patient in supine position.

_____ d. Bathe patient as necessary.

_____ e. Close patient's eyes and mouth if needed.

_____ f. Allow family to view body and remain in the room.

10. The patient asks the patient care technician what the criteria are for admission to hospice. What is the best response? (511–512)

1. "Hospice care is available to everyone regardless of sex, race, age, religion, diagnosis, or ability to pay."

2. "There must be a medical diagnosis of terminal cancer with poor prognosis for curative treatment."

3. "You and your primary caregiver must understand and be willing to participate in the planning of care."

4. "The whole family must be informed about life support measures and be willing to be involved in the decision-making."

11. The family of a dying patient is feeling physically and emotionally exhausted while taking shifts to care for their loved one 24 hours a day. This family could best benefit from the hospice service of: (514)

1. respite care.

2. palliative care consultation.

3. bereavement counseling.

4. the hospice ethics committee.

12. The hospice volunteer tells the patient care technician that he is thinking about quitting. "I like the patient, but the wife has me doing the shopping, the yardwork, and walking the dog. Now she wants me to paint the house." What should the patient care technician do? (514)

1. Talk to the wife and explain the role and responsibilities of the volunteer.

2. Call the volunteer coordinator and ask for additional help to paint the house.

3. Ask the patient how he has been getting along with the volunteer.

4. Instruct the volunteer to explain the situation to the volunteer coordinator.

CRITICAL THINKING ACTIVITY

13. The patient is an 86-year-old who has Alzheimer's disease. His 80-year-old wife has been taking care of him at home for the past 10 years. He was recently diagnosed with an aggressive and inoperable cancer. His family agrees that he should be in hospice, but they are unable to agree on who should be the primary caregiver. The wife insists that she has been taking care of her husband for 10 years and is capable. The eldest son has been responsible for paying the bills and overseeing his parents' finances; he thinks that his sister, who is a nurse but lives in a different state, should move back and be the caregiver. The sister thinks that the grandson who is living with his grandparents and attends the university should be the caregiver. The grandson agrees that he is at the house most often, but is reluctant to take the responsibility. Discuss how the hospice team can assist this family in the decision-making process. (Table 35.1 and 35.2)

_____

_____

_____

_____

_____

_____

_____

_____

_____

Procedures Checklists

These checklists were developed to assist in evaluating the competence of students in performing the interventions presented in *Fundamental Concepts and Skills for the Patient Care Technician*. Students can be evaluated with a "Satisfactory (S)" or an "Unsatisfactory (U)" performance rating by putting a check in the appropriate column for each step. Specific instruction or feedback can be provided in the "Comments" column. All the checklists have been streamlined to include **only** the critical steps needed to satisfactorily master the skill. They are **not** intended to replace the text, which describes and illustrates each skill in detail.

This page intentionally left blank

PROCEDURE 9-1

PERFORMING HAND HYGIENE WITH SOAP AND WATER

	S	U	Comments
1. Inspect hands, observing for visible soiling, breaks, or cuts in the skin and cuticles.	☐	☐	_____
2. Determine amount of contaminant on hands.	☐	☐	_____
3. Assess areas around the skin that are contaminated.	☐	☐	_____
4. Adjust the water to appropriate temperature and force.	☐	☐	_____
5. Wet hands and wrists under the running water, always keeping hands lower than elbows.	☐	☐	_____
6. Lather hands with liquid soap (about 1 teaspoon).	☐	☐	_____
7. Wash hands thoroughly with a firm, circular motion and friction on back of hands, palms, and wrists. Wash each finger individually, paying special attention to areas between fingers and knuckles by interlacing fingers and thumbs and moving hands back and forth, causing friction.	☐	☐	_____
8. Wash for 15 to 30 seconds.	☐	☐	_____
9. Rinse wrists and hands completely, again keeping hands lower than elbows.	☐	☐	_____
10. Dry hands thoroughly with paper towels. Start by patting at fingertips, then hands, and then wrists and forearms.	☐	☐	_____
11. If it is necessary to turn off faucets manually, use a dry paper towel.	☐	☐	_____
12. Use hospital-approved hand lotion if desired.	☐	☐	_____
13. Inspect hands and nails for cleanliness.	☐	☐	_____
14. If hands are not visibly soiled, use an alcohol-based waterless antiseptic for routine decontamination of hands in all clinical situations, unless you are caring for a patient with *Clostridium difficile* or Candida infection. The spores are unaffected by alcohol, so soap and water must be used in this instance.	☐	☐	_____
15. If contamination occurs, it is necessary to reassess technique.	☐	☐	_____

This page intentionally left blank

PROCEDURE 9-2

GLOVING

	S	U	Comments

Donning Gloves

1. Remove gloves from dispenser. ☐ ☐ _____

2. Inspect gloves for perforations. ☐ ☐ _____

3. Don gloves when ready to begin patient care. Wearing gloves with a gown does not necessitate any special technique for putting them on; wear them pulled over cuffs of gown. ☐ ☐ _____

4. Change gloves after direct handling of infectious material such as wound drainage. ☐ ☐ _____

5. Do not touch side rails, tables, or bed stands with contaminated gloves. ☐ ☐ _____

Removing Gloves

6. Remove first glove by grasping outer surface at palm with other gloved hand and pulling glove inside out and off. Place this glove in the hand that is still gloved. ☐ ☐ _____

7. Remove second glove by placing finger under cuff and turning glove inside out and over other glove. Drop gloves into waste container. ☐ ☐ _____

8. Perform hand hygiene. ☐ ☐ _____

9. If contamination occurs, it is necessary to reassess technique. ☐ ☐ _____

This page intentionally left blank

PROCEDURE 9-3

GOWNING FOR ISOLATION

	S	U	Comments
1. Push up long sleeves, if you have them.	☐	☐	_____
2. Perform hand hygiene.	☐	☐	_____
3. Don gown and tie it securely at neck and waist.	☐	☐	_____
4. Remove gown after providing necessary patient care.	☐	☐	_____
5. Discard soiled gown appropriately.	☐	☐	_____
6. Perform hand hygiene.	☐	☐	_____
7. Record use of gown in isolation procedure if required by the health care agency. Some agencies charge a daily rate for isolation precautions. This is noted on a daily basis in the patient's record. Therefore, repeated notations throughout the 24 hours are not necessary.	☐	☐	_____
8. If contamination occurs, it is necessary to reassess technique.	☐	☐	_____

This page intentionally left blank

PROCEDURE 9-4

DONNING A MASK

	S	U	Comments
1. Remove mask from container.	☐	☐	_____
2. Don mask when ready to begin patient care by covering your nose, mouth, and eyes (or glasses) with the device. Wear a mask with a protective eye shield when there is risk of splashing. Secure mask in place with elastic band or by tying the strings behind your head.	☐	☐	_____
3. Wear mask until it becomes moist, but no longer than 20 to 30 minutes.	☐	☐	_____
4. Remove mask by untying the strings or moving the elastic. Be certain not to touch contaminated area.	☐	☐	_____
5. Dispose of soiled mask in appropriate container.	☐	☐	_____
6. Wash hands thoroughly.	☐	☐	_____
7. Record use of mask during patient care (some agencies require documentation of specific barriers used).	☐	☐	_____
8. If contamination occurs, it is necessary to reassess technique.	☐	☐	_____

This page intentionally left blank

PROCEDURE 9-5

ISOLATION PRECAUTIONS

	S	U	Comments

1. Follow agency policy for specific type of transmission-based precautions used. ☐ ☐ _____

2. Ensure that the environment has the equipment and supplies for the type of isolation:

   a. Private or isolation room with anteroom ☐ ☐ _____

   b. Adequate hand hygiene facilities ☐ ☐ _____

   c. Containers for trash, soiled linen, and sharp instruments (such as needles) ☐ ☐ _____

3. Provide explanation of isolation precautions to patient, family, and visitors. ☐ ☐ _____

4. Post sign on door of patient's room or wall outside room stating the type of protective measures in use for patient care. ☐ ☐ _____

5. Be certain to supply the room with lined containers designated for soiled linens and for trash. ☐ ☐ _____

6. Assess vital signs with designated equipment if possible, administer medications, administer hygiene, and collect specimens. ☐ ☐ _____

7. Report any changes in patient's health status to nurse. ☐ ☐ _____

8. Record assessments and performance of transmission-based precautions. Document per agency policy. ☐ ☐ _____

9. Additional techniques for acid-fast bacillus (AFB) isolation (airborne precautions):

   a. Before entering room, don N-95 respirator mask that you have undergone a fit-test for. ☐ ☐ _____

   b. Record assessments and performance of patient care. ☐ ☐ _____

This page intentionally left blank

PROCEDURE 9-6

USING AN ALCOHOL-BASED WATERLESS ANTISEPTIC FOR ROUTINE HAND HYGIENE

	S	U	Comments
1. If hands are not visibly soiled, use an alcohol-based waterless antiseptic for routine decontamination of hands in most clinical situations.	☐	☐	_____
2. Apply an ample amount of product to palm of one hand.	☐	☐	_____
3. Rub hands together, covering all surfaces of hands and fingers with antiseptic.	☐	☐	_____
4. Rub hands together for several seconds until alcohol is dry.	☐	☐	_____
5. Allow hands to dry before applying gloves.	☐	☐	_____
6. If an adequate volume is used, 15 to 25 seconds are needed for hands to dry.	☐	☐	_____
7. If hands are dry or chapped, a small amount of facility-approved lotion or barrier cream can be applied.	☐	☐	_____

This page intentionally left blank

PROCEDURE 9-7

PREPARING A STERILE FIELD

	S	U	Comments
1. Prepare sterile field just before planned procedure. Be sure to use supplies immediately.	☐	☐	_____
2. Select clean work surface that is above waist level.	☐	☐	_____
3. Assemble necessary equipment.	☐	☐	_____
4. Check dates, labels, and condition of package for sterility of equipment.	☐	☐	_____
5. Wash hands thoroughly.	☐	☐	_____
6. Place package containing sterile drape on work surface and open.	☐	☐	_____
7. With fingertips of one hand, pick up folded top edge of sterile drape.	☐	☐	_____
8. Gently lift drape up from its outer cover and let it unfold by itself without touching any object. Discard outer cover with your other hand.	☐	☐	_____
9. With other hand, grasp adjacent corner of drape and hold the entire edge straight up and away from your body. Now, properly place drape while using two hands and being sure to keep the drape away from nonsterile surfaces.	☐	☐	_____
a. Holding drape, first position the bottom half over intended work surface.	☐	☐	_____
b. Allow top half of drape to be placed over work surface last.	☐	☐	_____
10. Perform procedure using sterile technique.	☐	☐	_____

This page intentionally left blank

PROCEDURE 9-8

PERFORMING OPEN STERILE GLOVING

	S	U	Comments

1. Have package of properly sized sterile gloves at treatment area. ☐ ☐ _____

2. Perform thorough hand hygiene. ☐ ☐ _____

3. Remove outer glove package wrapper by carefully separating and peeling apart sides. ☐ ☐ _____

4. Grasping inner side of package, lay package on clean, flat surface just above waist level. Open package, keeping gloves on wrapper's inside surface. ☐ ☐ _____

5. Identify right and left gloves. Each glove has a cuff approximately 2 inches (5 cm) deep. ☐ ☐ _____

6. Glove dominant hand first. With thumb and first two fingers of nondominant hand, grasp edge of cuff of glove for dominant hand. Touch only glove's inside surface. ☐ ☐ _____

7. Carefully pull glove over dominant hand, leaving cuff; be sure cuff does not roll up wrist. Be sure thumb and fingers are in proper spaces. ☐ ☐ _____

8. With gloved dominant hand, slip fingers underneath second glove's cuff in such fashion that the cuff will protect the gloved fingers. ☐ ☐ _____

9. Carefully pull second glove over nondominant hand. Do not allow fingers and thumb of gloved dominant hand to touch any part of exposed nondominant hand. Keep thumb of dominant hand abducted back. ☐ ☐ _____

10. After second glove is on, interlock hands. Be sure to touch only sterile sides. The cuffs usually fall down after application. ☐ ☐ _____

Glove Removal and Disposal

11. Grasp outside of one cuff with other gloved hand; avoid touching wrist. ☐ ☐ _____

12. Pull glove off, turning it inside out. Discard in receptacle. ☐ ☐ _____

13. Take fingers of bare hand and tuck inside remaining glove cuff. Peel glove off, inside out. Discard in receptacle. ☐ ☐ _____

121

This page intentionally left blank

PROCEDURE 9-9

OPENING AND POURING A STERILE SOLUTION

	S	U	Comments
1. Verify the expiration date of the sterile solution prior to opening.	☐	☐	_____
2. Open the cap or lid to the bottle, taking great care not to touch the inside of the bottle cap or the inside of the bottle.	☐	☐	_____
3. After removing the cap or lid, either hold it in your hand or place it sterile side up (inside up), on a clean surface.	☐	☐	_____
4. Hold the bottle with the label in the palm of the hand to prevent the solution from wetting the label.	☐	☐	_____
5. Keep the edge of the bottle from touching the edge of the receiving container.	☐	☐	_____
6. Pour the solution slowly to avoid splashing the underlying drape or sterile field.	☐	☐	_____
7. Hold the bottle over the outside edge of the sterile field.	☐	☐	_____

This page intentionally left blank

Student Name_____ Date_____

PROCEDURE 12-1

POSITIONING PATIENTS

	S	U	Comments
1. Assemble equipment and supplies:			
Pillows	☐	☐	_____
Footboard	☐	☐	_____
Trochanter roll	☐	☐	_____
Splinting devices	☐	☐	_____
Hand rolls	☐	☐	_____
Safety reminder devices	☐	☐	_____
Side rails	☐	☐	_____
2. Request assistance as needed.	☐	☐	_____
3. Introduce self.	☐	☐	_____
4. Identify patient.	☐	☐	_____
5. Explain procedure.	☐	☐	_____
6. Perform hand hygiene. Wear gloves as necessary according to agency policy and guidelines from the Centers for Disease Control and Prevention (CDC) and Occupational Safety and Health Administration (OSHA).	☐	☐	_____
7. Prepare patient.	☐	☐	_____
8. Close door or pull curtain.	☐	☐	_____
9. Raise level of bed to comfortable working height.	☐	☐	_____
10. Remove pillows and devices used in previous position.	☐	☐	_____
11. Put bed in flat position, or as low as patient can tolerate, and lower side rail closest to you.	☐	☐	_____
12. Position patient:			
a. Dorsal (supine) position:			
(1) Place patient on back with head of bed flat.	☐	☐	_____
(2) Place small rolled towel under lumbar area of back.	☐	☐	_____

125

	S	U	Comments

(3) Place pillow under upper shoulder, neck, and head. ☐ ☐ _____

(4) Place trochanter rolls parallel to lateral surface of thighs. ☐ ☐ _____

(5) Place small pillow or roll under ankle to elevate heels. ☐ ☐ _____

(6) Support feet in dorsiflexion with firm pillow, footboard, or high-top sneakers. ☐ ☐ _____

(7) Place pillows under pronated forearms, keeping upper arms parallel to patient's body. ☐ ☐ _____

(8) Place hand rolls in patient's hands. ☐ ☐ _____

b. Dorsal recumbent position (supine position with patient lying on back, head, and shoulder with extremities moderately flexed; legs are sometimes extended):

(1) Move patient and mattress to head of bed. ☐ ☐ _____

(2) Turn patient onto back. ☐ ☐ _____

(3) Assist patient to raise legs, bend knees, and allow legs to relax. ☐ ☐ _____

(4) Replace pillow. Patient sometimes needs a small lumbar pillow. ☐ ☐ _____

c. Fowler's position:

(1) Move patient and mattress to head of bed. ☐ ☐ _____

(2) Raise head of bed to 45 to 60 degrees. ☐ ☐ _____

(3) Replace pillow. ☐ ☐ _____

(4) Use footboard or firm pillow. ☐ ☐ _____

(5) Use pillows to support arms and hands. ☐ ☐ _____

(6) Place small pillow or roll under ankles. ☐ ☐ _____

d. Semi-Fowler's position:

(1) Move patient and mattress to head of bed. ☐ ☐ _____

(2) Raise head of bed to about 30 degrees. ☐ ☐ _____

(3) Replace pillow. ☐ ☐ _____

e. Orthopneic position (often used for the patient with a cardiac or respiratory condition):

	S	U	Comments
(1) Elevate head of bed to 90 degrees. Patient sometimes sits on side of bed with legs dangling or propped on a chair.	☐	☐	_____
(2) Place pillow between patient's back and mattress.	☐	☐	_____
(3) Place pillow on overbed table and assist patient to lean over, placing head on pillow.	☐	☐	_____

f. Sims' position (the left Sims' position is appropriate positioning for the enema procedure and administration of a rectal suppository): ☐ ☐ _____

(1) Place patient in supine position.	☐	☐	_____
(2) Position patient in lateral position, lying partially on the abdomen.	☐	☐	_____
(3) Draw knee and thigh up near abdomen and support with pillows.	☐	☐	_____
(4) Place patient's lower arm along the back.	☐	☐	_____
(5) Bring upper arm up, flex elbow, and support with pillow.	☐	☐	_____
(6) Allow patient to lean forward to rest on chest.	☐	☐	_____

g. Prone position:

(1) Assist patient onto abdomen with face to one side.	☐	☐	_____
(2) Flex arms toward the head.	☐	☐	_____
(3) Position pillows for comfort. Place a pillow under lower leg to release any "pull" on the lower back, or place a pillow under the head (or both).	☐	☐	_____

h. Knee-chest (genupectoral) position: ☐ ☐ _____

(1) Turn patient onto abdomen.	☐	☐	_____
(2) Assist patient into kneeling position; arms and head rest on pillow while upper chest rests on bed.	☐	☐	_____

i. Lithotomy position: ☐ ☐ _____

(1) Position patient to lie supine (lying on the back).	☐	☐	_____
(2) Request patient to slide buttocks to edge of examining table.	☐	☐	_____

127

	S	U	Comments

(3) Lift both legs; have patient bend knees and place feet in stirrups. ☐ ☐ _____

(4) Drape patient. ☐ ☐ _____

(5) Provide small lumbar pillow if desired. ☐ ☐ _____

j. Trendelenburg's position:

(1) Place patient's head lower than body, with body and legs elevated and on an incline. Foot of bed is sometimes elevated on blocks. (Not used if patient has head or foot injury.) Trendelenburg's position was once used in the treatment of shock but is not used as frequently for this now because it causes pressure on the diaphragm by organs in the abdomen and shunts more blood to the brain rather than all of the vital organs. Trendelenburg's position is sometimes used to assist in venous distention during central line placement. ☐ ☐ _____

13. Ensure the patient is in proper body alignment. ☐ ☐ _____

14. Provide comfort by performing a back massage after turning from one position to another. ☐ ☐ _____

15. Reposition debilitated, unconscious, or paralyzed patients at least every 2 hours. ☐ ☐ _____

16. Perform hand hygiene. ☐ ☐ _____

17. Document. ☐ ☐ _____

PROCEDURE 12-2

PERFORMING RANGE-OF-MOTION EXERCISES

	S	U	Comments
1. Refer to medical record or care plan for special interventions.	☐	☐	_____
2. Assemble equipment: Clean gloves, if necessary	☐	☐	_____
3. Introduce self.	☐	☐	_____
4. Identify patient.	☐	☐	_____
5. Explain procedure.	☐	☐	_____
6. Perform hand hygiene and don clean gloves according to agency policy and guidelines from CDC and OSHA.	☐	☐	_____
7. Prepare patient for intervention:			
a. Close door to room or pull curtain.	☐	☐	_____
b. Drape for procedure if appropriate.	☐	☐	_____
c. Raise bed to comfortable working level.	☐	☐	_____
d. Assist patient to a comfortable position, either sitting or lying down.	☐	☐	_____
8. Support the body part above (proximal to) and below (distal to) the joint by cradling the extremity or by using cupped hand to support the joint being exercised.	☐	☐	_____
9. Begin by doing exercises in normal sequence. Repeat each full sequence five times during the exercise period. Discontinue exercise if patient reports pain or if resistance or muscle spasm occurs.	☐	☐	_____
10. Assist patient by putting each joint through full range of motion.	☐	☐	_____
11. Position patient for comfort. To prevent contracture (an abnormal shortening of a muscle), do not allow patients with joint pain to remain continuously in position of comfort; joints must be exercised routinely. Periodically provide back massage.	☐	☐	_____
12. Adjust bed linen.	☐	☐	_____
13. Remove and dispose of gloves and wash hands.	☐	☐	_____
14. Document the following:			

Procedures Checklists

	S	U	Comments
Joints exercised	☐	☐	_____
Presence of edema or pressure areas	☐	☐	_____
Any discomfort resulting from the exercises	☐	☐	_____
Any limitations of ROM	☐	☐	_____
Patient's tolerance of the exercises	☐	☐	_____

PROCEDURE 12-3

MOVING THE PATIENT

	S	U	Comments
1. Refer to the medical record or care plan for special interventions.	☐	☐	_____
2. Assemble equipment:			
Hospital bed	☐	☐	_____
Chair	☐	☐	_____
Side rails	☐	☐	_____
Patient's slippers	☐	☐	_____
Cotton blanket	☐	☐	_____
Pillows	☐	☐	_____
Extra personnel	☐	☐	_____
Lifting devices (see Procedure 12.4)	☐	☐	_____
3. Introduce self.	☐	☐	_____
4. Identify patient.	☐	☐	_____
5. Explain procedure.	☐	☐	_____
6. Perform hand hygiene.	☐	☐	_____
7. Prepare patient for intervention:			
a. Close door or pull curtain.	☐	☐	_____
b. Adjust bed level to safe working height.	☐	☐	_____
8. Arrange for assistance as necessary.	☐	☐	_____
9. Lift and move patient up in bed:			
a. Place patient supine with head flat.	☐	☐	_____
b. Face the patient and establish base of support.	☐	☐	_____
c. Use a lift (draw) sheet to assist patient up in bed.	☐	☐	_____
(1) Roll patient first to one side and then the other, placing lift sheet underneath patient from shoulders to thighs.	☐	☐	_____

	S	U	Comments

(2) Flex knees and face body in the direction of the move. The foot farthest away from the bed faces forward for broader base of support. ☐ ☐ _____

(3) With one staff member on each side of patient, grasp lift sheet firmly with hands near patient's upper arms and hips, rolling the sheet material until hands are close to the patient. ☐ ☐ _____

(4) Instruct patient to rest arms over body and to lift head on the count of 3; at the same time, pull the sheet to move the patient up to head of bed. ☐ ☐ _____

10. Turning the patient:

a. Stand with feet slightly apart and flex knees. ☐ ☐ _____

b. If the patient is unable to assist in turning, two people should use the lift sheet to turn the patient. ☐ ☐ _____

c. Move patient's body to one side of the bed. ☐ ☐ _____

d. If patient is assisting in turning, turn the patient on side facing raised side rail, toward the patient care technician. If patient is not assisting, then use the lift sheet to turn the patient. ☐ ☐ _____

e. Flex one of patient's legs over the other. Place pad or pillow between legs. ☐ ☐ _____

f. Align patient's shoulders; place pillow under head. ☐ ☐ _____

g. Support patient's back with pillows as necessary. A "tuck back" pillow is made by folding pillow lengthwise. Tuck smooth area slightly under patient's back. ☐ ☐ _____

11. Dangling patient:

a. Assess pulse and respirations. ☐ ☐ _____

b. Move patient to side of bed toward the patient care technician. ☐ ☐ _____

c. Lower bed to lowest position. ☐ ☐ _____

d. Raise head of bed. ☐ ☐ _____

e. Support patient's shoulders and help to swing legs around and off bed; do this all in one motion by simply pivoting patient. Ensure patient's feet touch floor. ☐ ☐ _____

	S	U	Comments

f. Another way to accomplish this is by rolling the patient onto his or her side before sitting the patient up. The patient care technician then stoops and, when standing, brings the patient along with the patient care technician. ☐ ☐ _____

g. Help patient place slippers on; cover legs. For safety, have patient place slippers on while in bed. ☐ ☐ _____

h. Assess patient's pulse and respirations. ☐ ☐ _____

12. Log-rolling the patient:

   a. Enlist the help of at least one additional person. ☐ ☐ _____

   b. Lower the head of the bed as much as the patient can tolerate. ☐ ☐ _____

   c. Place a pillow between the patient's legs. Use of a pull sheet placed between shoulders and knees facilitates turning. ☐ ☐ _____

   d. Extend the patient's arm over the patient's head unless shoulder movement is restricted. If shoulder movement is restricted, keep the arm in extension next to the body. ☐ ☐ _____

   e. With two assistive staff on the same side of the bed, one of the staff places one hand on the patient's shoulder and the other on the hip, while the other staff places one hand to support the patient's back and the other behind the knee. If a lift sheet is used, space hands in such a way to provide even support for the length of the rolled sheet and to distribute weight evenly. ☐ ☐ _____

   f. On a count of 3, turn the patient with a continuous, smooth, and coordinated effort. ☐ ☐ _____

   g. Support the patient with pillows as previously discussed. ☐ ☐ _____

13. Transferring the patient from bed to straight chair or wheelchair:

   a. Lower bed to lowest position. ☐ ☐ _____

   b. Raise head of bed. ☐ ☐ _____

   c. Support patient's shoulders and help swing legs around and off bed; perform all in one motion. ☐ ☐ _____

   d. Help patient don robe and slippers. ☐ ☐ _____

	S	U	Comments

e. Have chair positioned beside bed with seat facing foot of bed. ☐ ☐ _____

  (1) Place wheelchair at right angle to bed and lock wheels after bed is lowered. ☐ ☐ _____

  (2) Place straight chair against wall or have another staff member hold the chair. ☐ ☐ _____

f. Stand in front of patient and place hands at patient's waist level or below; allow patient to use his or her arms and shoulder muscles to push down on the mattress to facilitate the move. ☐ ☐ _____

g. Assist patient to stand and swing around with back toward seat of chair. Keep the strong side toward the chair. ☐ ☐ _____

h. Help patient to sit down as the staff member bends his or her knees to assist process. ☐ ☐ _____

i. Apply blanket to legs. ☐ ☐ _____

j. If transfer belt is used, apply after patient is sitting on side of bed and follow these guidelines:

  (1) Stand in front of patient. ☐ ☐ _____

  (2) Have patient hold on to the mattress, or ask patient to place his or her fists on the bed by the thighs. ☐ ☐ _____

  (3) Be sure patient's feet are flat on the floor. ☐ ☐ _____

  (4) Have patient lean forward. ☐ ☐ _____

  (5) Instruct patient to place his or her hands on the PCT's shoulders, not around the PCT's neck or at the side. ☐ ☐ _____

  (6) Grasp the transfer belt at each side. ☐ ☐ _____

  (7) Brace knees against patient's knees. Block patient's feet with PCT's feet. ☐ ☐ _____

  (8) Ask patient to push down on the mattress and to stand on the count of 3. Pull patient into a standing position as you straighten your knees. ☐ ☐ _____

  (9) Pivot patient so he or she is able to grasp the far arm of the chair. Back of the legs will be touching the chair. ☐ ☐ _____

  (10) Continue to turn patient until the other arm rest is grasped. ☐ ☐ _____

	S	U	Comments

(11) Gradually lower patient into the chair as you bend your hips and knees. The patient assists if able by leaning forward and bending his or her elbows and knees. ☐ ☐ _____

(12) Ensure buttocks are to the back of the chair. ☐ ☐ _____

(13) Cover patient's lap and legs. ☐ ☐ _____

14. Transferring from bed to stretcher then back to bed:

    a. Position bed flat and raise to the same height as stretcher. Lower side rails. ☐ ☐ _____

    b. Cover patient with top sheet or blanket and remove linens without exposing patient. ☐ ☐ _____

    c. Assess for IV line, Foley catheter, tubes, or surgical drains, and position them to avoid tension during the transfer. ☐ ☐ _____

    d. Position the stretcher as close to the bed as possible, and lock the wheels of the bed and stretcher (with side rails lowered). ☐ ☐ _____

    e. When patient is able to assist, stand near side of stretcher and instruct patient to move feet, then buttocks, and finally upper body to the stretcher, bringing blanket along. Be certain patient's body is centered on the stretcher. ☐ ☐ _____

    f. When patient is unable to assist, place a folded sheet or bath blanket under patient so that it supports patient's head and extends to mid-thighs. Roll the sheet or bath blanket close to the patient's body. Assist patient to cross arms over chest. Two assistive staff reach over the bed to patient, and two more stand as close to the stretcher as possible. A fifth person stands at the foot to transfer the feet. Using a coordinating count of 3, all five staff lift the patient to the edge of the bed. With another effort, lift the patient from edge of bed to stretcher. Roller devices are available in some facilities to facilitate this transfer. ☐ ☐ _____

15. Transferring from bed to stretcher back to bed:

    a. Adjust the height of the bed to the level of the seat of the wheelchair if possible. ☐ ☐ _____

    b. Position the wheelchair at a 45-degree angle next to the bed. ☐ ☐ _____

	S	U	Comments
c. Face the wheelchair toward the foot of the bed midway between the head and foot of the bed.	☐	☐	_____
d. Lock the wheelchair. Locks are located above the rims of the wheels. Push handle forward to lock.	☐	☐	_____
e. Raise the footplates, and place the transfer belt on patient (if not already in place).	☐	☐	_____
f. Assist patient to move to the front of the wheelchair.	☐	☐	_____
g. Position yourself slightly in front of patient to guard and protect patient throughout the transfer.	☐	☐	_____
h. Coordinate transfer to the bed by having patient stand and then pivot to the side of the bed. Then have patient sit on the side of the mattress.	☐	☐	_____
i. With patient sitting on side of the bed, place your arm near the head of the bed under theperson's shoulders while supporting thehead and neck. Take your other arm andplace it under the person's knees. Bend yourknees and keep your back straight.	☐	☐	_____
j. Tell patient to help lift the legs when youbegin to move. On a count of 3, standing with a wide base of support, raisepatient's legs as you pivot his or her bodyand lower the shoulders onto the bed. Remember to keep your back straight.	☐	☐	_____
16. Perform hand hygiene.	☐	☐	_____
17. Assess patient for appropriate body alignment after move. When repositioning, always assess previously dependent skin surfaces (pressure areas). Position pillowsfor comfort. Do not overtire patient duringambulation. As in all transfers, be certain calldevice is in easy reach.	☐	☐	_____
18. Document procedure.	☐	☐	_____

PROCEDURE 12-4

USING LIFTS FOR MOVING PATIENTS

	S	U	Comments
1. Refer to medical record or care plan for special interventions. Read manual for direction.	☐	☐	_____
2. Assemble equipment:			
Mechanical lift frame	☐	☐	_____
Seat sling attachment (may be one piece or two) or a standing frame	☐	☐	_____
Two cotton bath blankets	☐	☐	_____
3. Introduce self.	☐	☐	_____
4. Identify patient.	☐	☐	_____
5. Explain procedure.	☐	☐	_____
6. Perform hand hygiene.	☐	☐	_____
7. Prepare patient for intervention:			
a. Close door or pull curtains.	☐	☐	_____
b. Adjust bed level to working height (even with level of arm of chair [of lift] if chair is not removable or level with seat if chair is removable).	☐	☐	_____
c. Place cotton bath blanket over chair for patient's comfort.	☐	☐	_____
d. Cover patient with remaining bath blanket.	☐	☐	_____
8. Secure adequate number of personnel.	☐	☐	_____
9. Place chair near bed.	☐	☐	_____
10. Appropriately place canvas seat under patient; support head and neck.	☐	☐	_____
11. Slide horseshoe-shaped bar under bed on one side.	☐	☐	_____
12. Lower horizontal bar to level of sling.	☐	☐	_____
13. Fasten hooks on chain to openings in sling.	☐	☐	_____
14. Raise head of bed.	☐	☐	_____
15. Fold patient's arms over chest.	☐	☐	_____
16. Pump lift handle until patient is raised off bed.	☐	☐	_____

	S	U	Comments
17. With steering handle, pull lift off bed and down to chair.	☐	☐	_____
18. Release valve slowly to lift and lower patient toward chair.	☐	☐	_____
19. Close off valve and release straps.	☐	☐	_____
20. Remove straps and lift.	☐	☐	_____
21. Perform hand hygiene.	☐	☐	_____
22. Document procedure:			
Evaluate body alignment to help prevent skin impairment.	☐	☐	_____
Evaluate patient's response to movement to help determine patient's mobility potential.	☐	☐	_____

PROCEDURE 12-5

APPLYING SAFETY REMINDER DEVICES

	S	U	Comments
1. Refer to medical record, care plan, and Kardex. Review agency policy.	☐	☐	_____
2. Perform hand hygiene.	☐	☐	_____
3. Introduce self.	☐	☐	_____
4. Identify patient.	☐	☐	_____
5. Procedure:			
a. Explain procedure.	☐	☐	_____
b. Prepare for procedure by providing privacy and assembling necessary supplies.	☐	☐	_____
c. Receive instructions for application of a SRD from the nurse (a comprehensive nursing assessment of the patient's potential for injury and treatment in relation to the need for an SRD is crucial before applying SRD).	☐	☐	_____
6. Apply appropriate type of SRD:			
a. Wrist or ankle (extremity) SRD designed to immobilize one or more extremities:	☐	☐	_____
(1) If using Kerlix gauze, make a clove hitch by forming a figure 8 and picking up the loops.	☐	☐	_____
(2) Place gauze or padding around the extremity.	☐	☐	_____
(3) Slip the wrist(s) or ankle(s) through loops directly over the padding; if using a commercially made SRD, wrap the padded portion of the device around affected extremity, thread tie through slit in device, and fasten to second tie with a secure knot.	☐	☐	_____
(4) Secure ends of ties to the movable portion of the bed frame that moves with the patient when the bed is adjusted, not to side rails.	☐	☐	_____
(5) Leave as much slack as possible (1 to 2 inches).	☐	☐	_____
(6) Palpate pulses below the SRD.	☐	☐	_____

	S	U	Comments
b. Elbow SRD:	☐	☐	_____
(1) Place SRD over the elbow or elbows.	☐	☐	_____
(2) Wrap SRD(s) snugly, tying them at the top. For small infants, tie or pin SRDs to their shirts.	☐	☐	_____
c. Vest:			
(1) Apply device over the patient's gown.	☐	☐	_____
(2) Put vest on patient with V-shaped opening in the front.	☐	☐	_____
(3) Pull tie at end of vest flap across the chest and slip tie through slit on opposite side of vest.	☐	☐	_____
(4) Wrap the other end of the flap across patient and tie the straps to frame of bed or behind wheelchair. Use the quick-release knot.	☐	☐	_____
(5) With a proper fit, there is room for a fist in the space between the vest and the patient.	☐	☐	_____
d. Gait or safety reminder belts:			
(1) Apply belt over the patient's gown.	☐	☐	_____
(2) If patient is ambulating, place belt around the patient's waist. The belt usually has a buckle to secure the belt in place.	☐	☐	_____
(3) If the belt does not have a buckle, use a slip knot.	☐	☐	_____
7. Use a quick-release knot rather than a regular knot to secure the SRD to bed frame.	☐	☐	_____
8. Secure SRDs so that the patient cannot untie them.	☐	☐	_____
9. Apply SRD with gentleness and compassion.	☐	☐	_____
10. Perform hand hygiene.	☐	☐	_____
11. Document procedure:			
Reason(s) SRD needed	☐	☐	_____
If appropriate, the notification of the physician and time order obtained	☐	☐	_____
The time and type of SRD applied	☐	☐	_____
The ongoing assessment and monitoring of the patient's skin, extremity circulation, and mental status	☐	☐	_____
The response(s) of the patient	☐	☐	_____

	S	U	Comments

The periodic removal of the SRD and any skin care performed ☐ ☐ _____

If SRD removed, note time and follow-up assessments ☐ ☐ _____

If reapplication is needed, note reasons, time, and patient assessment ☐ ☐ _____

A flow sheet is an excellent tool for this documentation ☐ ☐ _____

12. Follow up:

    a. Monitor for skin impairment. ☐ ☐ _____

    b. With the use of extremity SRD, assess extremity distal to SRD every 30 minutes or more often according to agency policy. ☐ ☐ _____

      (1) Remove SRD on one extremity at a time at least every 2 hours for 5 minutes. ☐ ☐ _____

    c. Monitor position of SRD, circulation, skin condition, and mental status frequently. Remove SRD when no longer needed. ☐ ☐ _____

    d. With the use of vest SRD, monitor respiratory status. ☐ ☐ _____

    e. Do NOT leave the patient unattended during temporary removal of SRD. Do take advantage of removal to change patient's position and inspect skin. ☐ ☐ _____

    f. Gently massage the skin beneath SRD; apply lotion or powder if desired. ☐ ☐ _____

    g. Change SRD when soiled or wet. ☐ ☐ _____

    h. Assess frequently for tangled ties or pressure points from knots; adjust SRD device(s) as needed. ☐ ☐ _____

13. Evaluation:

    a. The SRD is adequate and appropriate for the individual patient's condition. ☐ ☐ _____

    b. SRDs are correctly applied. ☐ ☐ _____

    c. Quick-release knots are easily released. ☐ ☐ _____

    d. Related problems are identified. ☐ ☐ _____

14. Pediatric considerations:

    a. When a child must be restrained for a procedure, it is best that the person applying the restraint not be the child's parent or guardian. ☐ ☐ _____

	S	**U**	**Comments**

b. A mummy restraint is a safe, efficient, short-term method to restrain a small child or infant for examination or treatment.

(1) Open a blanket, and fold one corner toward the center. Place the infant on the blanket with shoulders at the fold and feet toward the opposite corner. ☐ ☐ _____

(2) With infant's right arm straight down against body, pull the right side of the blanket firmly across the right shoulder and chest, and secure beneath the left side of body. ☐ ☐ _____

(3) Place the left arm straight against the body, bring the left side of the blanket across the shoulder and chest, and lock beneath the infant's body on the right side. ☐ ☐ _____

(4) Align the infant's legs, pull the corner of the blanket near the feet up toward the body, and tuck snugly in place or fasten securely with safety pins. ☐ ☐ _____

15. Remain with the infant during restraint, and remove the restraint immediately after treatment is complete. If restraint is required for an extended period, remove it at least every 2 hours and perform range-of-motion exercises on all extremities. ☐ ☐ _____

PROCEDURE 12-6

ASSISTING WITH FALLS DURING AMBULATION

	S	U	Comments
1. Observe the patient closely.	☐	☐	_____
2. Encourage the patient to do the following:			
a. Take slow, deep breaths	☐	☐	_____
b. Keep eyes open and look straight ahead	☐	☐	_____
c. Keep head up	☐	☐	_____
3. If the patient starts to fall, do not attempt to prevent the fall. Ease the patient to the floor. This allows you to break the fall, control its direction, and also protect the patient's head.	☐	☐	_____
4. Follow these steps when assisting a patient's fall:	☐	☐	_____
a. Stand with your feet apart. Keep your back straight.	☐	☐	_____
b. Bring the patient close to your body as quickly as possible. Use the gait belt if one is worn. If not, wrap your arms around the patient's waist.	☐	☐	_____
c. Move your leg so the patient's buttocks rest on it.	☐	☐	_____
5. Move the leg near the patient.	☐	☐	_____
a. Lower the patient to the floor by letting the patient slide down your leg. Bend at your hips and knees as you lower the patient.	☐	☐	_____
b. Call for assistance.	☐	☐	_____
c. Return patient to bed.	☐	☐	_____
6. Report and document the following:	☐	☐	_____
a. How the fall occurred.	☐	☐	_____
b. How far the patient walked.	☐	☐	_____
c. How activity was tolerated before the fall.	☐	☐	_____
d. Any report of symptoms before the fall.	☐	☐	_____
e. The amount of assistance needed by the patient while walking.	☐	☐	_____
f. Complete an incident report, if required.	☐	☐	_____

This page intentionally left blank

PROCEDURE 13-1

MAINTAIN PROVIDER/PROFESSIONAL-LEVEL CPR CERTIFICATION: USE AN AUTOMATED EXTERNAL DEFIBRILLATOR*

	S	U	Comments
1. Place the AED near the victim's left ear. Turn on the AED.	☐	☐	_____
2. Attach electrode pads to the victim's bare dry chest as pictured on the AED.	☐	☐	_____
3. Place the electrodes at the sternum and apex of the heart.	☐	☐	_____
4. Make sure the pads are in complete contact with the victim's chest and that they do not overlap.	☐	☐	_____
5. All rescuers must clear away from the victim.	☐	☐	_____
6. Press the ANALYZE button.	☐	☐	_____
7. The AED analyzes the victim's coronary status, announces whether the victim is going to be shocked, and automatically charges the electrodes.	☐	☐	_____
8. All rescuers must clear away from the victim. Press the SHOCK button if the machine is not automated. You may repeat three analyze-shock cycles.	☐	☐	_____
9. Deliver one shock, leaving the AED attached, and immediately perform CPR, starting with chest compressions.	☐	☐	_____
10. After 2 minutes of CPR, repeat the AED analysis and deliver another shock, if indicated. If a nonshockable rhythm is detected, the AED should instruct the rescuer to resume CPR immediately, beginning with chest compressions.	☐	☐	_____
11. If the machine gives the "No Shock Indicated" signal, assess the victim. Check the carotid pulse and breathing status and keep the AED attached until EMS arrives. (Continue to monitor breathing and circulation, because these can stop at any time. Keep the AED pads in place to diagnose ventricular fibrillation quickly if it occurs.)	☐	☐	_____

_____

*These steps are to be performed only on an approved mannequin.

This page intentionally left blank

PROCEDURE 13-2

PERFORM FIRST AID PROCEDURES: CARE FOR A PATIENT WHO HAS FAINTED

	S	U	Comments

1. If warning is given that the patient feels faint, have the patient lower the head to the knees to increase the blood supply to the brain. If this does not stop the episode, have the patient lie down on the examination table or lower the patient to the floor. If the patient collapses to the floor when fainting, treat with caution because of possible head or neck injuries. ☐ ☐ _____

2. Immediately notify the physician of the patient's condition and assess the patient for life-threatening emergencies, such as respiratory or cardiac arrest. If the patient is breathing and has a pulse, monitor the patient's vital signs. ☐ ☐ _____

3. Loosen any tight clothing and keep the patient warm, applying a blanket if needed. ☐ ☐ _____

4. If a head or neck injury is not a factor, elevate the patient's legs above the level of the heart using the footstool with pillow support if available. (Elevating the legs assists with venous blood return to the heart. This may relieve symptoms of fainting by elevating the blood pressure and increasing blood flow to vital organs.) ☐ ☐ _____

5. Continue to monitor vital signs and apply oxygen by nasal cannula if ordered by the physician. ☐ ☐ _____

6. If vital signs are unstable or the patient does not respond quickly, activate emergency medical services (EMS).(Fainting may be a sign of a life-threatening problem.) ☐ ☐ _____

7. If the patient vomits, roll the patient onto his or her side to prevent aspiration of vomitus into the lungs. ☐ ☐ _____

8. Once the patient has completely recovered, assist the patient into a sitting position. Do not leave the patient unattended on the examination table. ☐ ☐ _____

This page intentionally left blank

PROCEDURE 13-3

MAINTAIN PROVIDER/PROFESSIONAL-LEVEL CPR CERTIFICATION: PERFORM ADULT RESCUE BREATHING, ONE-RESCUER AND TWO-RESCUER CPR; PERFORM PEDIATRIC AND INFANT CPR*

	S	U	Comments

To Perform One-Rescuer CPR on an Adult Victim

1. Establish unresponsiveness. Tap the victim and ask, "Are you OK?" Wait for the victim to respond. ☐ ☐ _____

2. Activate the emergency response system. Get the AED. Use your personal cell phone if nearby to avoid leaving the patient. Put on gloves and get a ventilator mask. [As soon as it is determined that an adult victim requires emergency care, activate emergency medical services (EMS). Most adults with sudden, nontraumatic cardiac arrest are in ventricular fibrillation. The time from collapse to defibrillation is the single most important predictor of survival.] ☐ ☐ _____

3. Tilt the victim's head by placing one hand on the forehead and applying enough pressure to push the head back; with the fingers of the other hand under the chin, lift up and pull the jaw forward. Look, listen, and feel for signs of breathing. Place your ear over the mouth and listen for breathing. Watch the rising and falling of the chest for evidence of breathing. ☐ ☐ _____

4. At the same time you are checking for breathing, check the patient's pulse (at the carotid artery for an adult or older child; at the brachial artery for an infant). If a pulse is present, continue rescue breathing (1 breath every 5 to 6 seconds—about 10 to 12 breaths per minute for an adult; 1 breath every 3 seconds—about 12 to 20 breaths per minute for an infant or child). If no signs of circulation are present, begin cycles of chest compressions at a rate of 100-120 compressions per minute for an adult followed by two slow breaths. ☐ ☐ _____

5. To deliver chest compressions, kneel at the victim's side a couple of inches away from the chest. Hand placement is over the sternum, between the nipples but above the xiphoid process. ☐ ☐ _____

149

	S	U	Comments

6. Place the heel of your hand on the chest over the lower part of the sternum. ☐ ☐ _____

7. Place your other hand on top of the first and interlace or lift your fingers upward off the chest. (This position gives you the most control, allowing you to avoid injuring the victim's ribs as you compress the chest.) ☐ ☐ _____

8. Bring your shoulders directly over the victim's sternum as you compress downward, keeping your elbows locked. ☐ ☐ _____

9. Depress the sternum at least 2 inches in an adult victim. Avoid pressing down more than 2.4 inches; injury can occur. Relax the pressure on the sternum after each compression but do not remove your hands from the sternum. (The depth of compression is needed to circulate blood through the heart. Movement of the hands may cause injury to the victim.) ☐ ☐ _____

10. After performing 30 compressions (at a rate of 100-120 compressions per minute), perform the head tilt–chin lift maneuver to open the airway, and give two rescue breaths. Each breath should only take 1 second. ☐ ☐ _____

11. Continue the cycle of 30 compressions to 2 breaths until help arrives, or an AED arrives. If the patient starts to respond with movement as well as a pulse and respiratory rate, move the patient to a recovery position. ☐ ☐ _____

Adult Two-Rescuer CPR

1. Rescuer 1 should check for a response from the person by asking "Are you okay?" ☐ ☐ _____

2. Rescuer 1 should check for breathing and a pulse for not more than 10 seconds. If there is no breathing or a pulse within the 10 seconds, CPR is begun. ☐ ☐ _____

3. Expose the person's chest and ensure he/she is in a supine position. ☐ ☐ _____

4. If the victim does not have a pulse, then the compressor begins to give chest compressions at a rate of 100-120 per minute. Count out loud so that you can establish a regular rhythm. Allow the chest to recoil between each compression. Give 30 compressions. ☐ ☐ _____

	S	U	Comments

5. Press down with each compression at least 2 inches but not more than 2.4 inches. Pressing down too far can cause injury to the patient. ☐ ☐ _____

6. Open the person's airway using the head tilt–chin lift method and give two rescue breaths. Each breath should not last longer than 1 second. The chest should rise and fall with each breath. ☐ ☐ _____

7. Continue the cycle of 30 compressions to 2 breaths, minimizing interruptions to no longer than 10 seconds. ☐ ☐ _____

8. Rescuer 2 obtains the AED, opens the case, and turns it on (See Procedure 13.1). Once the AED has performed an analysis, the AED will indicate whether or not a shock will be given. ☐ ☐ _____

9. Once the AED has given a shock, CPR will be resumed by Rescuers 1 & 2. One rescuer will give30 chest compressions; the other will give 2 rescue breaths. ☐ ☐ _____

10. When the AED signals for a rhythm check, pause and change positions. ☐ ☐ _____

11. Resume CPR after the rhythm check by giving 30 chest compressions and 2 rescue breaths. Continue with this pattern until the person begins to move or until a code team or Rapid Response Team arrives to provide advanced cardiac life support. If the person begins to move, position him/her in the recovery position. ☐ ☐ _____

To Perform CPR on a Child

The procedure for giving CPR to a child ages 1 through 8 is essentially the same as that for an adult. The differences are as follows:

1. Start CPR if the child's heart rate is less than 60 beats per minute. ☐ ☐ _____

2. Perform 5 cycles of compressions and breaths on the child (30:2 ratio, about 2 minutes) before calling 911 or the local emergency number or using an AED. If another person is available, have that person activate EMS while you care for the child. (It is important to provide immediate circulation of oxygenated blood to a child to prevent brain damage. Most pediatric cardiac arrests occur because of a secondary problem, such as airway occlusion, rather than a cardiac problem. If you know there is an airway obstruction, clear the obstruction and then proceed with CPR.) ☐ ☐ _____

151

	S	U	Comments

3. Use only one hand to perform chest compressions. (The pediatric sternum requires less force to achieve the needed depression.) □ □ _____

4. Breathe more gently. □ □ _____

5. When two rescuers are present, change the compression-to-breath ratio to 15 compressions to 2 breaths. For one rescuer, the same ratio for adults is used for children, 30 compressions followed by 2 breaths per cycle; after 2 breaths, immediately begin the next cycle of compressions and breaths. □ □ _____

6. Give only enough air to make the chest rise. □ □ _____

7. Chest compressions should compress about 1/3 of the depth, or 2 inches. □ □ _____

8. After 5 cycles (about 2 minutes) of CPR without response, use a pediatric AED if available. □ □ _____

9. Continue until the child responds or help arrives. □ □ _____

10. Infant cardiac arrest typically is caused by lack of oxygen from drowning or choking. If you know the infant has an airway obstruction, clear the obstruction; if you do not know why the infant is unresponsive, perform CPR for 2 minutes (about 5 cycles) before calling 911 or the local emergency number. □ □ _____

11. If another person is available, have that person call for help immediately while you attend to the baby. □ □ _____

Rescue Breathing for an Infant

1. Use an infant ventilator mask or cover the baby's mouth and nose with your mouth. □ □ _____

2. Give two rescue breaths by gently puffing out the cheeks and slowly breathing into the infant's mouth, taking about 1 second for each breath. □ □ _____

To Perform CPR on an Infant

1. For single rescuer CPR, draw an imaginary line between the infant's nipples. Place two fingers on the sternum just below this intermammary line. □ □ _____

2. For 2-rescuer CPR, use the two-thumb encircling hands method. □ □ _____

	S	U	Comments
3. Gently compress the chest 1.5 inches deep.	☐	☐	_____
4. Compression rate should be 100 to 120 per minute.	☐	☐	_____
5. Administer 2 breaths after every 30 compressions.	☐	☐	_____
6. After about five 30:2 cycles, activate EMS.	☐	☐	_____
7. Continue CPR until the infant responds or help arrives.	☐	☐	_____
8. Remove your gloves and the ventilator mask valve, and discard them in the biohazard container. Disinfect the ventilator mask per the manufacturer's recommendations. Sanitize your hands.	☐	☐	_____
9. Document the procedure and the patient's condition.	☐	☐	_____

_____

*These steps are to be performed only on an approved mannequin.

This page intentionally left blank

PROCEDURE 13-4

PERFORM FIRST AID PROCEDURES: RESPOND TO AN AIRWAY OBSTRUCTION CHOKING IN AN ADULT*

	S	U	Comments

1. Ask, "Are you choking?" If the victim indicates yes, ask, "Can you speak?" If the victim is unable to speak, tell the victim you are going to help. (If the victim is unable to speak, is coughing weakly, and/or is wheezing, he or she has an obstructed airway with poor air exchange, and the obstruction must be removed before respiratory arrest occurs.)   ☐ ☐ _____

2. Stand behind the victim with your feet slightly apart.   ☐ ☐ _____

3. Reach around the victim's abdomen and place an index finger into the victim's navel or at the level of the belt buckle. Make a fist of the opposite hand (do not tuck the thumb into the fist) and place the thumb side of the fist against the victim's abdomen above the navel. If the victim is pregnant, place the fist above the enlarged uterus. If the victim is obese, it may be necessary to place the fist higher in the abdomen. It may be necessary to perform chest thrusts on a victim who is pregnant or obese. (The fist should be placed in the soft tissue of the abdomen to avoid injury to the sternum or rib cage.)   ☐ ☐ _____

4. Place the opposite hand over the fist and give abdominal thrusts in a quick inward and upward movement. Repeat the abdominal thrusts until the object is expelled or the victim becomes unresponsive.   ☐ ☐ _____

Unresponsive Adult Victim

1. Carefully lower the patient to the ground, activate the emergency response system, and put on disposable gloves.   ☐ ☐ _____

2. Immediately begin cardiopulmonary resuscitation (CPR) with 30 compressions and 2 breath cycles using the ventilator mask. (Higher airway pressures are maintained with chest compressions than with abdominal thrusts.)   ☐ ☐ _____

	S	U	Comments

3. Each time the airway is opened to deliver a rescue breath during CPR, look for an object in the victim's mouth and remove it if visible. If no object is found, immediately return to the cycle of 30 chest compressions. ☐ ☐ _____

4. A finger sweep should be used only if the rescuer can see the obstruction. ☐ ☐ _____

5. Continue cycles of 30 compressions to 2 rescue breaths until the obstruction is removed or emergency medical services (EMS) arrives. ☐ ☐ _____

6. If the obstruction is removed, assess the victim for breathing and circulation. If a pulse is present but the patient is not breathing, begin rescue breathing. ☐ ☐ _____

7. Once the patient has been stabilized or EMS has taken over care, remove your gloves and the ventilator mask valve and discard them in the biohazard container. Disinfect the ventilator mask per the manufacturer's recommendations. Sanitize your hands. ☐ ☐ _____

8. Document the procedure and the patient's condition. ☐ ☐ _____

These steps are to be performed only on an approved mannequin.

PROCEDURE 13-5

PERFORM FIRST AID PROCEDURES: CONTROL BLEEDING

	S	U	Comments
1. Sanitize your hands and put on appropriate personal protective equipment.	☐	☐	_____
2. Assemble equipment and supplies.	☐	☐	_____
3. Apply several layers of sterile dressing material directly to the wound and exert pressure.	☐	☐	_____
4. Wrap the wound with bandage material. Add more dressing and bandaging material if the bleeding continues.	☐	☐	_____
5. If bleeding persists and the wound is on anextremity, elevate the extremity above the level of the heart. Notify the physician immediately if the bleeding cannot be controlled.	☐	☐	_____
6. If the bleeding still continues, maintain direct pressure and elevation; also apply pressure to the appropriate artery. If the bleeding is in the arm, apply pressure to the brachial artery by squeezing the inner aspect of the middle upper arm. If the bleeding is in the leg, apply pressure to the femoral artery on the affected side by pushing with the heel of the hand into the femoral crease at the groin. If the bleeding cannot be controlled, emergency medical services (EMS) may need to be activated.	☐	☐	_____
7. Once the bleeding has been brought under control and the patient has been stabilized, discard contaminated materials in an appropriate biohazard waste container.	☐	☐	_____
8. Disinfect the area, then remove your gloves and discard them in a biohazard waste container.	☐	☐	_____
9. Sanitize your hands.	☐	☐	_____
10. The nurse will document the incident, including details of the wound, when and how it occurred, the patient's symptoms and vital signs, treatment provided by the physician, and the patient's current condition.	☐	☐	_____

This page intentionally left blank

PROCEDURE 15-1

OBTAIN VITAL SIGNS: OBTAIN AN ORAL TEMPERATURE USING A DIGITAL THERMOMETER

	S	U	Comments
1. Sanitize your hands.	☐	☐	_____
2. Assemble the needed equipment and supplies.	☐	☐	_____
3. Identify the patient and explain the procedure. Make sure the patient has not eaten, consumed any hot or cold fluids, smoked, or exercised during the 30 minutes before the temperature is measured.	☐	☐	_____
4. Prepare the probe for use as described in the package directions. Make sure probe covers are always used.	☐	☐	_____
5. Place the probe under the patient's tongue and instruct the patient to close the mouth tightly without biting down on the thermometer. Help the patient by holding the probe end.	☐	☐	_____
6. When a beep is heard, remove the probe from the patient's mouth and immediately eject the probe cover into an appropriate biohazard waste container. Note the reading in the LED window of the processing unit.	☐	☐	_____
7. Record the reading in the patient's medical record.	☐	☐	_____
8. Sanitize your hands and disinfect the equipment as indicated.	☐	☐	_____

This page intentionally left blank

PROCEDURE 15-2

OBTAIN VITAL SIGNS: OBTAIN AN AURAL TEMPERATURE USING A TYMPANIC THERMOMETER

	S	U	Comments
1. Sanitize your hands.	☐	☐	_____
2. Gather the necessary equipment and supplies.	☐	☐	_____
3. Identify your patient and explain the procedure.	☐	☐	_____
4. Place a disposable cover on the probe.	☐	☐	_____
5. Follow the package directions to start the thermometer.	☐	☐	_____
6. Insert the probe into the ear canal far enough to seal the opening. Do not apply pressure. For children younger than age 3, gently pull the earlobe down and back; for patients older than age 3, gently pull the top of the ear up and back.	☐	☐	_____
7. Press the button on the probe as directed. The temperature will appear on the display screen in 1 to 2 seconds.	☐	☐	_____
8. Remove the probe, note the reading, and discard the probe cover into a biohazard container without touching it.	☐	☐	_____
9. Sanitize your hands and disinfect the equipment if indicated.	☐	☐	_____
10. Record the temperature results in the patient's medical record.	☐	☐	_____

This page intentionally left blank

Student Name_____ Date_____

PROCEDURE 15-3

OBTAIN VITAL SIGNS: OBTAIN A TEMPORAL ARTERY TEMPERATURE

	S	U	Comments
1. Sanitize your hands.	☐	☐	_____
2. Gather the necessary equipment and supplies.	☐	☐	_____
3. Introduce yourself, identify your patient, and explain the procedure.	☐	☐	_____
4. Remove the protective cap on the probe. The probe can be cleaned by lightly wiping the surface with an alcohol swab.	☐	☐	_____
5. Push the patient's hair up off of the forehead to expose the site. Gently place the probe on the patient's forehead, halfway between the eyebrows and the hairline.	☐	☐	_____
6. Depress and hold the SCAN button and lightly glide the probe sideways across the patient's forehead to the hairline just above the ear. As you move the sensor across the forehead, you will hear a beep, and a red light will flash.	☐	☐	_____
7. Keep the button depressed, lift the thermometer, and place the probe on the upper neck behind the ear lobe. The thermometer may continue to beep, indicating that the temperature is rising.	☐	☐	_____
8. When scanning is complete, release the button and lift the probe. Note the temperature recorded on the digital display. The scanner automatically turns off 15 to 30 seconds after release of the button.	☐	☐	_____
9. Disinfect the thermometer if indicated and replace the protective cap.	☐	☐	_____
10. Sanitize your hands.	☐	☐	_____
11. Record the temperature results in the patient's medical record.	☐	☐	_____

This page intentionally left blank

PROCEDURE 15-4

OBTAIN VITAL SIGNS: OBTAIN AN AXILLARY TEMPERATURE

	S	U	Comments
1. Sanitize your hands.	☐	☐	_____
2. Gather the necessary equipment and supplies.	☐	☐	_____
3. Introduce yourself, identify your patient, and explain the procedure.	☐	☐	_____
4. Prepare the thermometer or digital unit in the same manner as for oral use.	☐	☐	_____
5. Remove the patient's clothing and gown the patient as needed to access the axillary region.	☐	☐	_____
6. Pat the patient's axillary area dry with tissues if needed.	☐	☐	_____
7. Cover the thermometer or probe and place the tip into the center of the armpit, pointing the stem toward the upper chest, making sure the thermometer is touching only skin, not clothing.	☐	☐	_____
8. Instruct the patient to hold the arm snugly across the chest or abdomen until the thermometer beeps.	☐	☐	_____
9. Remove the thermometer, note the digital reading, and dispose of the cover in the biohazard waste container.	☐	☐	_____
10. Disinfect the thermometer if indicated.	☐	☐	_____
11. Sanitize your hands.	☐	☐	_____
12. Record the axillary temperature on the patient's medical record.	☐	☐	_____

This page intentionally left blank

PROCEDURE 15-5

OBTAIN VITAL SIGNS: OBTAIN AN APICAL PULSE

	S	U	Comments
1. Sanitize your hands and clean the stethoscope earpieces and diaphragm with alcohol swabs.	☐	☐	_____
2. Introduce yourself, identify your patient, and explain the procedure.	☐	☐	_____
3. If necessary, assist the patient in disrobing from the waist up and provide the patient with a gown that opens in the front.	☐	☐	_____
4. Assist the patient into the sitting or supine position.	☐	☐	_____
5. Hold the stethoscope's diaphragm against the palm of your hand for a few seconds.	☐	☐	_____
6. Place the stethoscope just below the left nipple in the intercostal space between the fifth and sixth ribs over the apex of the heart.	☐	☐	_____
7. Listen carefully for the heartbeat.	☐	☐	_____
8. Count the pulse for 1 full minute. Note any irregularities in rhythm and volume.	☐	☐	_____
9. Help the patient sit up and dress.	☐	☐	_____
10. Sanitize your hands.	☐	☐	_____
11. Record the pulse in the patient's chart and record any arrhythmias.	☐	☐	_____

This page intentionally left blank

PROCEDURE 15-6

OBTAIN VITAL SIGNS: ASSESS THE PATIENT'S RADIAL PULSE

	S	U	Comments
1. Sanitize your hands.	☐	☐	_____
2. Introduce yourself, identify your patient, and explain the procedure.	☐	☐	_____
3. Place the patient's arm in a relaxed position, palm downward, at or below the level of the heart.	☐	☐	_____
4. Gently grasp the palm side of the patient's wrist with your first three fingertips approximately 1 inch below the base of the thumb.	☐	☐	_____
5. Count the beats for 1 full minute using a watch with a second hand.	☐	☐	_____
6. Sanitize your hands.	☐	☐	_____
7. Record the count and any irregularities on the patient's medical record. The pulse usually is recorded immediately after the temperature.	☐	☐	_____

This page intentionally left blank

PROCEDURE 15-7

OBTAIN VITAL SIGNS: DETERMINE THE RESPIRATORY RATE

	S	U	Comments
1. Sanitize your hands.	☐	☐	_____
2. Introduce yourself and identify the patient.	☐	☐	_____
3. The patient's arm is in the same position used to count the pulse. If you have difficulty noticing the patient's breathing, place the arm across the chest to detect movement.	☐	☐	_____
4. Note the rise and fall of the patient's chest.	☐	☐	_____
5. Count the respirations for 30 seconds, using a watch with a second hand, and multiply by	☐	☐	_____
6. Release the patient's wrist.	☐	☐	_____
7. Sanitize your hands.	☐	☐	_____
8. Record the respirations on the patient's medical record after the pulse recording.	☐	☐	_____

This page intentionally left blank

PROCEDURE 15-8

OBTAIN VITAL SIGNS: DETERMINE A PATIENT'S BLOOD PRESSURE

	S	U	Comments

1. Sanitize your hands. ☐ ☐ _____

2. Assemble the equipment and supplies needed. Clean the earpieces and diaphragm of the stethoscope with alcohol swabs. ☐ ☐ _____

3. Introduce yourself, identify your patient, and explain the procedure. ☐ ☐ _____

4. Select the appropriate arm for application of the cuff (no mastectomy on that side, with out injury or disease). If the patient has had a bilateral mastectomy, the blood pressure should be taken using a large thigh cuff with the stethoscope over the popliteal artery. ☐ ☐ _____

5. Seat the patient in a comfortable position with the legs uncrossed and the arm resting palm up at heart level on the lap or a table. ☐ ☐ _____

6. Roll up the sleeve to about 5 inches above the elbow or have the patient remove the arm from the sleeve. ☐ ☐ _____

7. Determine the correct cuff size. ☐ ☐ _____

8. Palpate the brachial artery at the antecubital space in both arms. If one arm has a stronger pulse, use that arm. If the pulses are equal, select the right arm. ☐ ☐ _____

9. If a female patient has had a mastectomy, the blood pressure should never be taken on the affected side. Compressing the arm may cause complications. If she has had a bilateral mastectomy, another site such as the popliteal artery must be used, which requires use of a thigh cuff. ☐ ☐ _____

10. Center the cuff bladder over the brachial artery with the connecting tube away from the patient's body and the tube to the bulb close to the body. ☐ ☐ _____

11. Place the lower edge of the cuff about 1 inch above the palpable brachial pulse, normally located in the natural crease of the inner elbow, and wrap it snugly and smoothly. ☐ ☐ _____

12. Position the gauge of the sphygmomanometer so that it is easily seen. ☐ ☐ _____

S   **U**   **Comments**

13. Palpate the brachial pulse, tighten the screw valve on the air pump, and inflate the cuff until the pulse can no longer be felt. Make a note at the point on the gauge where the pulse could no longer be felt. Mentally add 30 mm Hg to the reading. Deflate the cuff and wait 15 seconds. ☐ ☐ _____

14. Insert the earpieces of the stethoscope turned forward into the ear canals. ☐ ☐ _____

15. Place the stethoscope's diaphragm over the palpated brachial artery for an adult patient or the bell for a pediatric patient. Press firmly enough to obtain a seal but not so tightly that the artery is constricted. ☐ ☐ _____

16. Close the valve and squeeze the bulb to inflate the cuff, rapidly but smoothly, to 30 mm Hg above the palpated pulse level, which was previously determined. ☐ ☐ _____

17. Open the valve slightly and deflate the cuff at a constant rate of 2 to 3 mm Hg per heartbeat. ☐ ☐ _____

18. Listen throughout the entire deflation; note the point on the gauge at which you hear the first sound (systolic) and the last sound (diastolic) until the sounds have stopped for at least 10 mm Hg. Read the pressure to the closest even number. ☐ ☐ _____

19. Do not reinflate the cuff once the air has been released. Wait 30 to 60 seconds to repeat the procedure if needed. ☐ ☐ _____

20. Remove the stethoscope from your ears and record the systolic and diastolic readings as BP systolic/diastolic. ☐ ☐ _____

21. It is recommended that the blood pressure be checked and recorded in each arm during the initial assessment of the patient and then bilaterally periodically after that for patients with hypertension. ☐ ☐ _____

22. Remove the cuff from the patient's arm and return it to its proper storage area. Clean the earpieces of the stethoscope with alcohol and return it to storage. ☐ ☐ _____

23. Sanitize your hands. ☐ ☐ _____

24. The provider may order the blood pressure recorded with the patient in two different positions to determine whether orthostatic hypotension is a factor. To perform this skill: ☐ ☐ _____

   a. Measure and record the patient's blood pressure (as detailed earlier) while the patient is either supine or sitting. ☐ ☐ _____

	S	U	Comments
b. Leave the cuff in place.	☐	☐	_____
c. Have the patient stand, and immediately measure the blood pressure again.	☐	☐	_____
d. Record the second blood pressure, as well as any patient symptoms, such as complaints of (c/o) vertigo or lightheadedness.	☐	☐	_____

This page intentionally left blank

PROCEDURE 15-9

ASSESSING OXYGEN SATURATION

	S	U	Comments

1. Determine the need to measure patient's oxygen saturation from the nurse or patient medical record. (Examples may include acute or chronic respiratory problems, chest wall injury, monitoring during unconscious sedation, and recovery from sedation or anesthesia.)   ☐ ☐ _____

2. Identify factors that influence measurement of SpO_2: oxygen therapy, respiratory therapy treatments such as postural drainage and percussion, hemoglobin level, hypotension, temperature, and medications such as bronchodilators.   ☐ ☐ _____

3. Review patient's medical record for health careprovider's order, or consult facility's proceduremanual for oxygen saturation measurementstandard of care.   ☐ ☐ _____

4. Determine previous baseline SpO_2 (if available) from patient's record.   ☐ ☐ _____

5. Determine most appropriate patient-specific site (e.g., finger, earlobe, bridge of nose, forehead) for sensor probe placement by measuring capillary refill. If capillary refill is greater than 2 seconds, select alternative site.   ☐ ☐ _____

   a. Site must have adequate local circulation and be free of moisture.   ☐ ☐ _____

   b. A finger free of polish or acrylic nail is preferred (Cicek et al., 2011).   ☐ ☐ _____

   c. If patient has tremors or is likely to move, use earlobe or forehead.   ☐ ☐ _____

   d. If patient is obese, clip-on probe may not fit properly; obtain a disposable(tape-on) probe.   ☐ ☐ _____

6. Position patient comfortably. Instruct patient to breathe normally. If the finger is the monitoring site, support lower arm.   ☐ ☐ _____

7. If using the finger, remove fingernail polish from digit with acetone or polish remover.   ☐ ☐ _____

8. Attach the sensor to monitoring site. Instruct patient that the clip-on probe will feel like a clothespin on the finger but will not hurt.   ☐ ☐ _____

	S	U	Comments

9. When the sensor is in place, turn on oximeter by activating power. Observe pulse waveform/intensity display and audible beep. Correlate oximeter pulse rate by taking patient's radial pulse. ☐ ☐ _____

10. Leave the sensor in place until oximeter readout reaches a constant value and pulse display reaches full strength during each cardiac cycle. Inform patient that the oximeter alarm will sound if the sensor falls off or if patient moves the sensor. Read SpO_2 on digital display. ☐ ☐ _____

11. If you are told to monitor oxygen saturation continuously, verify that SpO_2 alarm limits are preset by the manufacturer at a low of85% and a high of 100%. Determine limits for SpO_2 and pulse rate as indicated by patient's condition. Verify that alarms are on. Assess skin integrity under sensor probe every2 hours; relocate sensor at least every 4 hours and more frequently if skin integrity is altered or tissue perfusion is compromised. ☐ ☐ _____

12. If you plan on intermittent monitoring or spot-checking SpO_2, remove the probe and turn oximeter power off. Store the sensor inappropriate location. ☐ ☐ _____

13. Compare SpO_2 with patient's previous baseline and acceptable SpO_2 if indicated by the nurse. Note use of oxygen therapy, which can affect oxygen saturation. ☐ ☐ _____

PROCEDURE 15-10

OBTAIN VITAL SIGNS: MEASURE A PATIENT'S WEIGHT AND HEIGHT

	S	U	Comments
1. Sanitize your hands.	☐	☐	_____
2. Introduce yourself, identify your patient, and explain the procedure.	☐	☐	_____
3. If the patient is to remove his or her shoes for weighing, place a paper towel on the scale platform. The patient may be given disposable slippers to wear.	☐	☐	_____
4. Check to see that the balance bar pointer floats in the middle of the balance frame when all weights are at zero.	☐	☐	_____
5. Help the patient onto the scale. Make sure a female patient is not holding a purse and that a male or female patient has removed any heavy objects from pockets.	☐	☐	_____
6. Move the large weight into the groove closest to the patient's estimated weight. The grooves are calibrated in 50-lb increments. If you choose a groove that is more than the patient's weight, the pointer will immediately tilt to the bottom of the balance frame. You then must move it back one groove.	☐	☐	_____
7. While the patient is standing still, slide the small upper weight to the right along the pound markers until the pointer balances in the middle of the balance frame.	☐	☐	_____
8. Leave the weights in place.	☐	☐	_____
9. Ask the patient to stand up straight and to look straight ahead. On some scales, the patient may need to turn with the back to the scale.	☐	☐	_____
10. Adjust the height bar so that it just touches the top of the patient's head.	☐	☐	_____
a. Leave the elevation bar set but fold down the horizontal bar (to maintain the height recording while protecting the patient from possible injury).	☐	☐	_____
b. Assist the patient off the scale. Make sure all items that were removed for weighing are given back to the patient.	☐	☐	_____

	S	U	Comments
c. Read the weight scale. Add the numbers at the markers of the large and small weights and record the total to the nearest ¼ lb on the patient's medical record.	☐	☐	_____
d. Record the height. Read the marker at the movable point of the ruler and record the measurement to the nearest ¼ inch on the patient's medical record.	☐	☐	_____
e. Use the patient's weight and height to record the BMI if this is office procedure.	☐	☐	_____
f. Return the weights and the measuring bar to zero.	☐	☐	_____
11. Sanitize your hands.	☐	☐	_____
12. Record the results on the patient's medical record.	☐	☐	_____

PROCEDURE 15-11

MAINTAIN GROWTH CHARTS: MEASURING AN INFANT'S LENGTH AND WEIGHT

	S	U	Comments

Measuring an Infant's Length

1. Sanitize your hands, assemble the necessary equipment, and explain the procedure to the infant's caregiver. ☐ ☐ _____

2. Undress the infant. The diaper may be left on while the length is measured, but it must be removed before the infant is weighed. ☐ ☐ _____

3. Ask the caregiver to place the infant on his or her back on the examination table, which is covered with paper. If the table is a pediatric table with a headboard, ask the caregiver to hold the infant's head gently against the headboard while you straighten the infant's leg and note the location of the heel on the measurement area. If there is no headboard, ask the caregiver to gently hold the infant's head still while you draw a line on the paper at the back of the baby's head and at the heel after the leg is extended. ☐ ☐ _____

4. Measure the infant's length with the tape measure and record it. ☐ ☐ _____

5. Document the results in either inches or centimeters, depending on office policy, on the infant's growth chart, in the progress notes, and in the caregiver's record if requested. Complete the growth chart graph by connecting the dot from the last visit. ☐ ☐ _____

Weighing an Infant

1. Sanitize your hands, assemble the necessary equipment, and explain the procedure to the infant's caregiver. ☐ ☐ _____

2. Prepare the scale by sliding weights to the left; line the scale with disposable paper (reduces the risk of pathogen transmission). ☐ ☐ _____

3. Completely undress the infant, including removing the diaper. (Extra clothing or diapers will alter the weight, making it an inaccurate reading.) ☐ ☐ _____

181

	S	U	Comments

4. Place the infant gently on the center of the scale, keeping your hand directly above the infant's trunk for safety.
☐ ☐ _____

5. Slide the weights across the scale until balance is achieved. Attempt to read the infant's weight while he or she is still.
☐ ☐ _____

6. Return the weights to the far left of the scale and remove the baby. The caregiver can rediaper the baby while you discard the paper lining the scale. If the scale became contaminated during the procedure, follow Occupational Safety and Health Administration (OSHA) guidelines for use of gloves and disposal of contaminated waste. Disinfect the equipment according to the manufacturer's guidelines.
☐ ☐ _____

7. Sanitize your hands.
☐ ☐ _____

8. Document the results in either pounds or kilograms, depending on office policy, on the infant's growth chart, in the progress notes, and in the caregiver's record if requested. Complete the growth chart by connecting the dot from the last visit.
☐ ☐ _____

PROCEDURE 15-12

MAINTAIN GROWTH CHARTS: MEASURE THE CIRCUMFERENCE OF AN INFANT'S HEAD

	S	U	Comments
1. Sanitize your hands.	☐	☐	_____
2. Identify the patient. If he or she is old enough, gain the child's cooperation through conversation.	☐	☐	_____
3. Place an infant in the supine position, or the infant may be held by the parent. An older child may sit on the examination table.	☐	☐	_____
4. Hold the tape measure with the zero mark against the infant's forehead, slightly above the eyebrows and the top of the ears. Ask the parent for assistance if necessary.	☐	☐	_____
5. Bring the tape measure around the head, just above the ears, until it meets.	☐	☐	_____
6. Read to the nearest 0.01 cm or ¼ inch.	☐	☐	_____
7. Record the measurement on the growth chart and in the patient's medical record.	☐	☐	_____
8. Dispose of the tape measure.	☐	☐	_____
9. Sanitize your hands.	☐	☐	_____

Procedures Checklists

This page intentionally left blank

PROCEDURE 16-1

PERFORM ELECTROCARDIOGRAPHY: OBTAIN A 12-LEAD ECG

	S	U	Comments

1. Sanitize your hands.　☐　☐　_____

2. Explain the procedure to the patient.　☐　☐　_____

3. Ask the patient to disrobe to the waist (including the bra for women) and remove belts, jewelry, socks, stockings, or pantyhose as necessary. If the patient is already wearing a gown, ask that it be positioned so that it opens in the front.　☐　☐　_____

4. Position the patient supine on the examination table and drape appropriately.　☐　☐　_____

5. Turn on the machine to allow the stylus to warm up; this may not be necessary with newer machines.　☐　☐　_____

6. Label the beginning of the tracing paper with the patient's name, the date, the time, and the patient's current cardiovascular medications or enter this information into the machine.　☐　☐　_____

7. At each location where an electrode will be placed, clean the skin with an alcohol wipe.　☐　☐　_____

8. Apply the self-adhesive electrodes to clean, dry, fleshy areas of the extremities. Extremely hairy areas may need to be shaved to achieve adequate electrode attachment, or place a piece of tape over the electrode to make sure it is secure.　☐　☐　_____

9. Apply the self-adhesive electrodes to the clean areas on the chest.　☐　☐　_____

10. Carefully connect the lead wires to the correct electrode with the alligator clips on the end of each lead. Make sure the lead wires are not crossed.　☐　☐　_____

11. Press the AUTO button on the machine and run the ECG tracing. The machine automatically places the standardization at the beginning, and the 12 leads then follow in the three-channel matrix with a lead II rhythm strip across the bottom of the page.　☐　☐　_____

12. Watch for artifacts during the recording. If artifacts are present, make appropriate corrections and repeat the recording to get a clean reading.　☐　☐　_____

	S	U	Comments
13. Remove the lead wires from the electrodes and then remove the electrodes from the patient.	☐	☐	_____
14. Assist the patient with getting dressed as needed. Clean and return the ECG machine to its storage area.	☐	☐	_____
15. Place the ECG recording in the patient's medical record for provider review.	☐	☐	_____
16. Sanitize your hands.	☐	☐	_____
17. Document the procedure in the patient's medical record.	☐	☐	_____

PROCEDURE 17-1

ADMITTING A PATIENT

	S	U	Comments
1. Perform hand hygiene.	☐	☐	_____
2. Prepare the room before the patient arrives: care items in place, bed at proper height and open, light on.	☐	☐	_____
3. Courteously greet the patient and family. Introduce yourself. Project interest and concern. Introduce roommate.	☐	☐	_____
4. Check the ID band and verify its accuracy.	☐	☐	_____
5. Assess immediate needs for toileting.	☐	☐	_____
6. Orient the patient to the unit, the lounge, and the nurses' station.	☐	☐	_____
7. Orient the patient to the room. Explain the use of equipment, call system, bed, telephone, and television.	☐	☐	_____
8. Explain facility routines, such as visiting hours and meal times.	☐	☐	_____
9. Provide privacy if the patient desires or if abuse is suspected. Family members are sometimes asked to leave the room. Admission of an infant or small child requires emotional support for both child and parents. Parents are generally encouraged to stay with their child to prevent separation anxiety. The most reliable source of admission information is the parent. Assist the patient to undress if necessary.	☐	☐	_____
10. Follow facility policy for care of valuables, clothing, and medications.	☐	☐	_____
11. Provide for safety: bed in low position, side rails up (unless admission is to a long-term care facility), call light within easy reach.	☐	☐	_____
12. Begin care as ordered by the nurse.	☐	☐	_____
13. Invite family back into the room if they left earlier.	☐	☐	_____
14. Perform hand hygiene.	☐	☐	_____
15. Record the information on the patient's health care record according to agency policy.	☐	☐	_____
16. Allow patient and family time alone together, if desired.	☐	☐	_____

This page intentionally left blank

PROCEDURE 17-2

TRANSFERRING A PATIENT

	S	U	Comments
1. Perform hand hygiene.	☐	☐	_____
2. Check health care provider's order for transfer and receive instruction from nurse.	☐	☐	_____
3. Inform patient and family of the transfer.	☐	☐	_____
4. Notify the receiving unit of the transfer and when to expect the patient.	☐	☐	_____
5. Gather all of the patient's belongings and necessary care items to accompany the patient.	☐	☐	_____
6. Assist in transferring the patient, usually via stretcher or wheelchair. The nurse will tell you how to transfer the patient.	☐	☐	_____
7. Introduce patient and family to nurses on new unit and to roommate.	☐	☐	_____
8. Perform hand hygiene.	☐	☐	_____
9. Record means of transfer. The nurse on the new unit also records an assessment of the patient's condition on arrival.	☐	☐	_____
10. For an intraagency transfer, other departments such as diagnostic imaging, laboratory, admission department, physical therapy, dietary, and business offices must be notified of the transfer.	☐	☐	_____
11. An interagency transfer is usually made via air or ground ambulance or via private car. Be sure the patient is dressed or covered appropriately for environmental comfort. If oxygen is necessary, a small transport tank is usually used. A nurse generally accompanies a critically ill patient who is being transferred.	☐	☐	_____
12. Infants are generally transported in an Isolette that is later returned to the sending health care facility. Parents usually accompany their child during transfer unless the transfer is via air ambulance. In this case, the parents generally follow in family transportation.	☐	☐	_____

This page intentionally left blank

PROCEDURE 17-3

DISCHARGING A PATIENT

	S	U	Comments
1. Perform hand hygiene.	☐	☐	_____
2. Be certain there is a discharge order.	☐	☐	_____
3. Notify the family or the person who will be transporting the patient home.	☐	☐	_____
4. Verify that the patient and the family or caregiver understand the instructions for care from the nurse.	☐	☐	_____
5. Gather equipment, supplies, and prescriptions that the patient is to take home.	☐	☐	_____
6. Assist the patient in dressing and packing items to go home.	☐	☐	_____
7. Check clothing and valuables list made on admission according to policy.	☐	☐	_____
8. Transfer the patient and belongings to the vehicle outside.			
a. Many facilities escort the patient via wheelchair.	☐	☐	_____
b. Many patients are discharged via stretcher.	☐	☐	_____
c. Assist the patient into the vehicle. Help the family place personal belongings into car. As with all procedures, use good communication skills and wish patients well as they leave the facility.	☐	☐	_____
9. Perform hand hygiene.	☐	☐	_____
10. Report to the nurse the time the patient was taken out of the facility and using what method (wheelchair, etc). Document the following:	☐	☐	_____
a. If the patient is an infant or child, they may be required to have a child restraint or car seat. This is determined by the state, and varies across states. If the family does not have an appropriate car seat, report this to the nurse before taking the patient off the unit.	☐	☐	_____

This page intentionally left blank

PROCEDURE 18-1

BATHING THE PATIENT AND ADMINISTERING A BACK RUB

	S	U	Comments
1. Refer to medical record, nurse, care plan, or Kardex for special interventions.	☐	☐	_____
2. Assemble the necessary supplies.			
3. Introduce self.	☐	☐	_____
4. Identify patient.	☐	☐	_____
5. Explain procedure to patient.	☐	☐	_____
6. Perform hand hygiene and, as appropriate, don clean gloves. Know agency policy and guidelines from the Centers for Disease Control and Prevention (CDC) and Occupational Safety and Health Administration (OSHA).	☐	☐	_____
7. Prepare patient for intervention:			
a. Close door or pull curtain.	☐	☐	_____
b. Drape for procedure as appropriate.	☐	☐	_____
c. Suggest use of bedpan, urinal, or bathroom.	☐	☐	_____
d. Arrange supplies.	☐	☐	_____
e. Adjust room temperature.	☐	☐	_____
f. Raise bed to comfortable working position.	☐	☐	_____
8. Bed bath:			
a. Lower side rail; position patient on side of bed closest to you.	☐	☐	_____
b. Loosen top linens from the foot of the bed; place bath blanket over the top linens. Ask patient to hold bath blanket while you remove top linens. If patient is unable, you need to hold bath blanket in place while removing linens.	☐	☐	_____
c. Place soiled laundry in laundry bag; do not touch uniform with soiled laundry.	☐	☐	_____
d. Assist patient with oral hygiene. If patient is unable, the nurse performs the procedure.	☐	☐	_____

	S	U	Comments

e. Remove patient's gown, all undergarments, and jewelry. If an extremity is injured or has reduced mobility, begin removal of the gown from the unaffected side. If the patient has an IV tube, remove gown from the arm without IV first, then lower IV container or remove tubing from pump and slide gown covering down over the affected arm and over tubing and container. Rehang IV container and check flow rate or reset pump. Do not disconnect tubing. ☐ ☐ _____

f. Raise side rail and fill washbasin two-thirds full with water at 110° F to 115° F (43° C to 46° C). To prevent spillage, do not overfill basin. ☐ ☐ _____

g. Remove pillow and raise head of bed to semi-Fowler's position if patient is able to tolerate it. ☐ ☐ _____

h. Form mitt with bath cloth around your hand; dip mitt and hand into bath water. Squeeze out excess water. ☐ ☐ _____

i. Wash around patient's eyes, using a different portion of washcloth for each eye. Cleanse from inner to outer canthus. Dry gently. ☐ ☐ _____

j. Rinse bath cloth (then continue to use as mitt) and finish washing face. Wash ears and neck. Cleanse pinna (the projecting part of the external ear) with cotton-tipped applicators. ☐ ☐ _____

k. Expose arm farthest from you. Place towel lengthwise under patient's arm. To cleanse the hands, the nurse can place washbasin on towel and place patient's hand in basin of water, or the hands can be cleansed with the washcloth (be sure to clean between the fingers). Bathe arms with long, firm strokes; a firm stroke rather than a light stroke prevents tickling the patient. Supporting arm, raise it above patient's head to bathe the axilla (the underarm area or armpit). Rinse and dry well. In most cases, provide nail care at this time (see next step), although if desired, it is possible to do separately. Apply deodorant if desired. ☐ ☐ _____

l. Bathe arm closest to you. Follow step k. ☐ ☐ _____

m. Cover patient's chest with bath towel; fold bath blanket down to waist and wash chest with circular motion. Be certain to cleanse and dry well in skin folds and under breasts. Continue to observe the condition of the patient's skin, degree of mobility, and behavior and encourage the patient to verbalize concerns. ☐ ☐ _____

	S	U	Comments

n. Fold bath blanket down to pubic area, keeping chest covered with dry towel. Wash abdomen, including umbilicus, and skin folds. Dry thoroughly. ☐ ☐ _____

o. Raise side rail; empty basin into hopper or stool. ☐ ☐ _____

p. Rinse basin and washcloth. Refill basin two-thirds full with water at 110° F to 115° F (43° C to 46° C). ☐ ☐ _____

q. Expose leg farthest away from you, keeping perineum covered. Place bath towel lengthwise on bed under patient's leg. Place washbasin on towel and place patient's foot in basin. Patients with diabetes mellitus need special foot care. Be certain to support patient's leg properly; flex knee and grasp heel. If patient is unable to place foot in washbasin, wash leg and foot with mitted washcloth. ☐ ☐ _____

r. With long firm strokes, bathe the leg. However, note that bathing the lower extremities of patients with history of deep vein thrombosis (DVT) or hypercoagulation disorders with long firm strokes is contraindicated; use circular, gentle strokes for these patients so that the clot is not dislodged. After soaking, do nail care. If skin is dry, apply lotion if desired. Do not massage legs. Never massage lower extremities. ☐ ☐ _____

s. Bathe leg and foot closest to you as in steps q and r. ☐ ☐ _____

t. Raise side rail. Be sure patient is covered with bath blanket. Be certain to expose only those body parts being bathed. Change water. Lower side rail. If patient tolerates, position prone or in Sims' position. Place towel lengthwise on bed along back. Wash and dry back from neckline down to buttocks. If patient tolerates a massage action, do so while washing back. ☐ ☐ _____

u. Reposition patient supine. Provide basin of water, soap, washcloth, and towel, and instruct patient to cleanse perineal area. If patient is unable to finish bath, don new gloves and complete this aspect of patient care. ☐ ☐ _____

v. Be certain patient is covered with blankets. Raise side rail. Empty, wash, and rinse basin. Replace basin in bedside stand. Place washcloth in laundry bag for soiled linen. ☐ ☐ _____

w. Position patient in Sims' or prone position close to you. Place towel lengthwise along patient's back. Give back rub. Never massage reddened areas. ☐ ☐ _____

	S	**U**	**Comments**

x. Assist patient into clean gown. If ordered, assist patient to ambulate to chair; place towel over shoulders, and comb hair. Women sometimes wish to apply makeup at this time. While patient is in chair, make unoccupied bed. If patient is not ambulatory, you have to make the occupied bed. ☐ ☐ _____

y. Place all soiled linen into laundry bag. Be certain all bath equipment is clean and put it away as necessary. ☐ ☐ _____

z. Place call light, overbed table, nightstand, and telephone within easy reach. ☐ ☐ _____

aa. Position patient for comfort, and provide warmth. ☐ ☐ _____

bb. Remove gloves, if wearing any; discard them in proper receptacle, and perform hand hygiene. Maintain a neat, clean work area. ☐ ☐ _____

9. The partial bed bath differs from the bed bath only in that the patient does not need assistance bathing many anatomic regions. Help by bathing those areas that the patient cannot reach (e.g., feet, back, perineal area). All steps of the bath are followed, and the same considerations prevail. Place supplies within easy reach. Change water as noted in the bed bath procedure, and give back care, skin care, nail care, and hair care. A partial bath, in which face, neck, hands, axilla, and perineum are washed, is practiced in some agencies. The feet might be included in a partial bed bath if necessary. ☐ ☐ _____

10. Towel bath*:

   a. Prepare patient:

   (1) Remove patient's clothing and excess bedding. Place patient on bath blanket, and cover patient with bath blanket. ☐ ☐ _____

   (2) Cover with plastic any surgical dressings, casts, or areas that are not to be gotten wet. ☐ ☐ _____

   (3) Fan fold a clean bath blanket at foot of the bed. ☐ ☐ _____

   (4) Position patient supine with legs partially separated and arms loosely at sides. ☐ ☐ _____

   b. Prepare towel:

   (1) Fold towel in half, top to bottom; fold in half again, top to bottom; fold in half again, side to side. Then roll towel–bath towel with bath towel and washcloths inside, beginning with folded edge. ☐ ☐ _____

	S	U	Comments

(2) Place rolled-up towel–bath towel in plastic bag with selvage edges toward open end of bag. ☐ ☐ _____

(3) Draw 2000 mL of water at 115° F to 120° F (46° C to 49° C) into plastic pitcher. If the towel is not warm, the sauna-like effect is not produced and the patient is chilled. Measure 30 mL of concentrate with a pump. Mix 2000 mL of water and no-rinse solution. ☐ ☐ _____

(4) Pour mixture over towel in plastic bag. ☐ ☐ _____

(5) Knead the solution quickly into towel; position plastic bag with open end in sink and squeeze out excess water. ☐ ☐ _____

c. Bathe patient with the following procedure:

(1) Fold bath blanket down to waist. Remove warm moist towel from plastic bag and place on patient's right or left chest with open edges up and outward. Unroll towel across chest. ☐ ☐ _____

(2) Open towel to cover entire body while removing top bath blanket. Tuck towel–bath towel in and around body. ☐ ☐ _____

(3) Begin bathing at feet, with gentle massaging motion. Use clean section of towel for each part of body as you move toward patient's head. ☐ ☐ _____

(4) Fold lower part of towel upward away from feet as bathing continues. If you have an assistant, the bath is given more effectively. ☐ ☐ _____

(5) Continue to draw clean bath blanket upward and place over patient as you move upward. Leave 3 inches of exposed skin between towel and bath blanket. Skin dries in 2 or 3 seconds. If towel bath is given properly, the patient is refreshed and relaxed. ☐ ☐ _____

(6) Wash face, neck, and ears with one of the prepared washcloths. ☐ ☐ _____

(7) Turn patient onto side. ☐ ☐ _____

(8) Use prepared bath towel for back care. ☐ ☐ _____

(9) Use second washcloth for perineal care (don disposable gloves). Sometimes you need a basin of warm water, soap, washcloth, towel, and gloves to perform perineal care. ☐ ☐ _____

(10) When bath is completed, remove towel and place with soiled linens in plastic laundry bag. ☐ ☐ _____

	S	U	Comments

(11) If top bath blanket is not soiled, fold for reuse later. □ □ _____

d. Make occupied bed. □ □ _____

11. Tub bath or shower:

a. Follow steps 1 and 3 to 7. □ □ _____

b. Determine whether activity is allowed by consulting patient's activity order. □ □ _____

c. Be certain tub or shower appliance is clean. See agency policy. Place nonskid mat on tub or shower floor if necessary and disposable mat outside of tub or shower. □ □ _____

d. Assemble all items necessary for bathing.

e. Assist patient to tub or shower. Shower chairs are available in most facilities to transport patients from the bedside to the shower, bathe and dry patients, and return them to bed. Be certain patient wears robe and slippers. □ □ _____

f. Instruct patient on how to use call signal. Place "in use" sign on tub or shower door if not using private bath. □ □ _____

g. If tub is used, fill with warm water, 109.4° F (43° C). Have patient test water if able, then adjust temperature. Instruct patient on use of faucets—which is hot and which is cold. If shower is used, turn water on and adjust temperature. □ □ _____

h. Caution patient to use safety bars. Discourage use of bath oil in water. Safety must be maintained at all times. Check on patient every 5 minutes. Do not allow to remain in tub more than 20 minutes. □ □ _____

i. Return when patient signals. Make an unoccupied bed while the patient bathes unless patient condition is such that you are required to remain with the patient. Return to the tub or shower room and offer to wash the patient's back. Knock before entering. □ □ _____

j. Assist patient out of tub and with drying. Observe the patient for signs and symptoms of weakness, such as rapid pulse, paleness, diaphoresis, unsteady gait, tachypnea, vertigo, and syncope. If patient reports weakness, vertigo, or syncope, drain tub before patient gets out and place towel over patient's shoulders. Notify the nurse. □ □ _____

	S	U	Comments

k. Assist patient into clean gown, robe, and slippers. Accompany to room, position for comfort, and give back rub. ☐ ☐ _____

l. Make unoccupied bed if patient can tolerate sitting in chair. Perform back, hair, nail, and skin care. ☐ ☐ _____

m. Return to shower or tub. Clean according to agency policy. Place all soiled linens in laundry bag and return all articles to patient's bedside. ☐ ☐ _____

n. Perform hand hygiene. ☐ ☐ _____

12. Tepid sponge bath for temperature reduction:

a. Follow steps 1 and 3 to 7. ☐ ☐ _____

b. Assess patient for elevated temperature. ☐ ☐ _____

c. Explain procedure to patient; outline steps of the procedure. ☐ ☐ _____

d. Assemble equipment. ☐ ☐ _____

e. Cover patient with bath blanket, remove gown, and close windows and doors. ☐ ☐ _____

f. Test water temperature. Place washcloths in water, then apply wet cloths to each axilla and groin. If patient is in tub, allow to stay in water for 20 to 30 minutes. ☐ ☐ _____

g. Gently sponge an extremity for about 5 minutes. If patient is in tub, gently sponge water over upper torso, chest, and back. ☐ ☐ _____

h. Continue sponge bath to other extremities and back for 3 to 5 minutes each. Assess temperature and pulse every 15 minutes. ☐ ☐ _____

i. Change water and reapply freshly moistened washcloths to axilla and groin as necessary. ☐ ☐ _____

j. Continue with sponge bath until body temperature falls to slightly above normal. Keep body parts that are not being sponged covered. Discontinue procedure according to agency policy. ☐ ☐ _____

k. Dry patient thoroughly and cover with light blanket or sheet. Avoid rubbing the skin too vigorously because that may cause an increase in heat production. Leave patient in comfortable position. ☐ ☐ _____

	S	U	Comments

l. Clean and return equipment to storage, clean area, and change bed linens as necessary. Perform hand hygiene. ☐ ☐ _____

13. Back rub:

a. Prepare supplies: ☐ ☐ _____

Bath blanket (optional) ☐ ☐ _____

Bath towel ☐ ☐ _____

Skin lotion, powder (if powder is used, apply sparingly) ☐ ☐ _____

b. Follow steps 1 and 3 to 7 and provide quiet environment. ☐ ☐ _____

c. Lower side rail. Position patient with back toward you. Cover patient so that only parts to massage are exposed. ☐ ☐ _____

d. Warm hands if necessary. Warm lotion by holding some in hands. Explain that lotion often feels cool. ☐ ☐ _____

e. Begin massage by starting in sacral area using circular motions. Stroke upward to shoulders. Massaging over bony prominences is no longer recommended because this may cause skin breakdown. ☐ ☐ _____

f. Use firm, smooth strokes to massage over scapulae. Continue to upper arms with one smooth stroke and down along side of back to iliac crest. Do not break contact with patient's skin. Complete massage in 3 to 5 minutes. ☐ ☐ _____

g. Gently but firmly knead skin by grasping area between thumb and fingers. Work across each shoulder and around nape of neck. Continue downward along each side to sacrum. ☐ ☐ _____

h. With long smooth strokes, end massage, remove excess lubricant from patient's back with towel, and retie gown. Position for comfort. Lower bed and raise side rail as needed and place call button within easy reach. ☐ ☐ _____

i. Place soiled laundry in proper receptacle, and perform hand hygiene. ☐ ☐ _____

14. Document:

Type of bath, water temperature, and solution used, when appropriate ☐ ☐ _____

	S	U	Comments
Duration of treatment	☐	☐	_____
Level of assistance required	☐	☐	_____
Vital signs, if applicable	☐	☐	_____
Patient's response	☐	☐	_____

15. Report alterations in skin integrity to nurse in charge or health care provider. ☐ ☐ _____

---

*An alternative to the towel bath is "bath-in-a-bag." This is similar to the towel bath except the washcloth is presoaked with no-rinse soap. The bag is placed in a warmer, and the patient is bathed. Some facilities use disposable cloths for bath-in-a-bag.

This page intentionally left blank

PROCEDURE 18-2

PERINEAL CARE: MALE AND FEMALE AND THE CATHETERIZED PATIENT

	S	U	Comments
1. Refer to medical record, care plan, or Kardex for special interventions.	☐	☐	_____
2. Assemble supplies.	☐	☐	_____
3. Introduce self.	☐	☐	_____
4. Identify patient.	☐	☐	_____
5. Explain procedure.	☐	☐	_____
6. Examine patient for the following, wearing gloves when in contact with mucous membranes or secretions:	☐	☐	_____
Accumulated secretions	☐	☐	_____
Surgical incision	☐	☐	_____
Lesions	☐	☐	_____
Ability to perform self-care	☐	☐	_____
Extent of care required by patient	☐	☐	_____
7. Remove and dispose of soiled gloves and perform hand hygiene and don clean gloves according to agency policy and guidelines from the CDC and OSHA.	☐	☐	_____
8. Prepare patient for interventions. Allow postpartum patients to perform this procedure by themselves while sitting on the stool, using a pericare squeeze bottle. Patients allowed tub or shower baths do this by themselves. Be certain supplies are close by.	☐	☐	_____
a. Close door or pull privacy curtain.	☐	☐	_____
b. Raise bed to comfortable working height and lower side rail.	☐	☐	_____
c. Arrange supplies at bedside.	☐	☐	_____
d. Assist patient to desired position in bed: dorsal recumbent for female or supine for male.	☐	☐	_____
e. Drape for procedure.	☐	☐	_____
9. Female perineal care:	☐	☐	_____

	S	U	Comments

a. Raise side rail and fill basin two-thirds full of water at 105° F to 109° F (41° C to 43° C). ☐ ☐ _____

b. Position waterproof pad or towel under patient's buttocks with patient lying in the dorsal recumbent position in bed. Drape patient with bath blanket placed in the shape of a diamond. One corner is under the patient's chin; one corner is on each side of the patient, with the bath blanket wrapped around each foot and leg; and the last corner is between the patient's legs. This corner can be lifted to expose the patient's perineum. ☐ ☐ _____

c. With a washcloth or disposable washcloth wrapped around one hand, wash and dry patient's upper thighs. ☐ ☐ _____

d. Wash both labia majora and labia minora. Wash carefully in skin folds. Cleanse in direction anterior to posterior. Use separate corner of washcloth for each skin fold. ☐ ☐ _____

e. Separate labia to expose the urinary meatus and the vaginal orifice. Wash downward toward rectum with smooth strokes. Use separate corner of washcloth for each smooth stroke. ☐ ☐ _____

f. Cleanse, rinse, and dry thoroughly. ☐ ☐ _____

g. Assist patient to side-lying position and cleanse rectal area with toilet tissue, if necessary. Wash area by cleansing from perineal area toward anus. You may often need several washcloths. Many facilities have disposable wipes. If so, use them. Wash, rinse, and dry thoroughly. ☐ ☐ _____

10. Male perineal care.

a. Raise side rail and fill basin two-thirds full of water at about 105° F to 109° F (41° C to 43° C). ☐ ☐ _____

b. Gently grasp shaft of penis. Retract foreskin of uncircumcised patient. ☐ ☐ _____

c. Wash tip of penis with circular motion. ☐ ☐ _____

d. Cleanse from meatus outward. Two washcloths are often necessary. Wash, rinse, and dry gently. ☐ ☐ _____

e. Replace foreskin, and wash shaft of penis with a firm but gentle downward stroke. Replace the foreskin of the uncircumcised male patient after thorough cleansing. ☐ ☐ _____

f. Rinse and dry thoroughly. ☐ ☐ _____

	S	U	Comments
g. Cleanse scrotum gently. Cleanse carefully in underlying skin folds. Rinse and dry gently.	☐	☐	_____
h. Assist patient to a side-lying position. Cleanse anal area. Follow step 9 g of female perineal care.	☐	☐	_____
11. Remove gloves. Clean and store equipment. Dispose of contaminated supplies in proper receptacle. Perform hand hygiene.	☐	☐	_____
12. Position patient for comfort.	☐	☐	_____
13. Document: Procedure	☐	☐	_____
Pertinent observations such as character and amount of discharge and odor if present, and patient's ability to perform own care	☐	☐	_____
14. Report abnormal findings to nurse in charge or health care provider.	☐	☐	_____

This page intentionally left blank

PROCEDURE 18-3

ADMINISTERING ORAL HYGIENE

	S	U	Comments
1. Refer to medical record, care plan, or Kardex for special interventions.	☐	☐	_____
2. Assemble supplies.			
3. Introduce self.	☐	☐	_____
4. Identify patient.	☐	☐	_____
5. Explain procedure to patient.	☐	☐	_____
6. Perform hand hygiene and don clean gloves according to agency policy and guidelines from the CDC and OSHA.	☐	☐	
7. Prepare patient for intervention:			
a. Close door or pull privacy curtain.	☐	☐	_____
b. Raise bed to comfortable working position.	☐	☐	_____
c. Arrange supplies.	☐	☐	_____
d. If patient tolerates the activity, provide supplies in the bathroom and allow patient privacy.	☐	☐	_____
e. If patient is on bed rest but tolerates the activity while remaining in bed, arrange overbed table in front of patient; provide supplies, and allow patient privacy.	☐	☐	_____
f. If you are performing the procedure with an unconscious patient, position patient's head to the side toward you and close to you.	☐	☐	_____
8. Oral care:			
a. Place towel under patient's face and emesis basin under patient's chin.	☐	☐	_____
b. Carefully separate patient's jaws.	☐	☐	_____
c. Cleanse mouth using brush, tongue blade, or Toothette moistened with cleansing agent. Clean inner and outer tooth surfaces. Swab roof of mouth and inside cheeks. Use flashlight for better visualization of oral cavity. Gently swab tongue. Rinse and repeat. Rinse several times.	☐	☐	
d. Apply lubricant to lips.	☐	☐	_____

This page intentionally left blank

PROCEDURE 18-4

DENTURE CARE

	S	U	Comments
1. Fill emesis basin half-full of tepid water or place a washcloth in the bottom of the sink.	☐	☐	_____
2. Ask patient to remove dentures and place in emesis basin. If patient is unable to remove own dentures, break suction that holds upper denture in place by using thumb and finger. With gauze, apply gentle downward tug and carefully remove from patient's mouth. Next, remove lower denture by carefully lifting up and turning sideways. Remove and place in emesis basin.	☐	☐	_____
3. Cleanse biting surfaces. Cleanse outer and inner tooth surfaces. Be certain to cleanse lower surface of dentures.	☐	☐	_____
4. Rinse dentures thoroughly with tepid water.	☐	☐	_____
5. Before replacing dentures in patient's mouth or after storing dentures properly, gently brush patient's gums, tongue, and inside of cheeks and rinse thoroughly.	☐	☐	_____
6. Replace dentures either in patient's mouth or in container of solution placed in safe place.	☐	☐	_____
7. When reinserting the dentures, replace the upper denture first if patient has both dentures. Apply gentle pressure to reestablish the suction. Moisten dentures for easier insertion. Be certain dentures are comfortably situated in patient's mouth before leaving the bedside.	☐	☐	_____
8. Dispose of gloves in proper receptacle. Clean and store supplies. Perform hand hygiene.	☐	☐	_____
9. Position patient for comfort, raise side rail, and lower bed.	☐	☐	_____
10. Assess for patient comfort.	☐	☐	_____
11. Document:			
Procedure	☐	☐	_____
Pertinent observations	☐	☐	_____
Most facilities have flow sheets for documenting activities of daily living (ADLs), but also note condition of oral cavity in nursing notes	☐	☐	_____
12. Report bleeding or presence of lesions to nurse in charge or to health care provider.	☐	☐	_____

209

This page intentionally left blank

PROCEDURE 18-5

BED MAKING

	S	U	Comments

1. Refer to medical record, nurse, care plan, or Kardex to determine potential for orders or specific precautions for mobility and positioning. ☐ ☐ _____

2. Gather supplies. ☐ ☐ _____

3. Introduce self. ☐ ☐ _____

4. Identify patient. ☐ ☐ _____

5. Explain procedure. ☐ ☐ _____

6. Perform hand hygiene and don gloves according to agency policy and guidelines from the CDC and OSHA. ☐ ☐ _____

7. Prepare patient:

   a. Close door or pull privacy curtain. ☐ ☐ _____

   b. Raise bed to appropriate height and lower side rail on the side closest to you. ☐ ☐ _____

   c. Lower head of bed (HOB) if patient tolerates it. ☐ ☐ _____

   d. Assess patient's tolerance of procedure. Be alert for signs of discomfort and fatigue. ☐ ☐ _____

8. Occupied bed:

   a. Remove spread and blanket separately and, if soiled, place in laundry bag. If linens will be reused, fold neatly and place over back of chair. Do not fan or shake linens. ☐ ☐ _____

   b. Place bath blanket over patient on top of sheet. ☐ ☐ _____

   c. Request patient to hold onto bath blanket while you remove top sheet by drawing sheet out from under bath blanket at foot of bed. If patient is unable to assist, you need to hold bath blanket in place while removing sheet. ☐ ☐ _____

   d. Place soiled sheet in laundry bag. ☐ ☐ _____

   e. With assistance from coworker, slide mattress to top of bed. ☐ ☐ _____

   f. Position patient to far side of bed with the back toward you. Assure patient that he or she will not fall out of bed. Adjust pillow for comfort. Be sure side rail is up. ☐ ☐ _____

211

	S	U	Comments

g. Beginning at head and moving toward foot, loosen bottom linens. Fan fold linen draw sheet, protective draw sheet, and bottom sheet, tucking edges of linens under patient. ☐ ☐ _____

h. Apply clean linens to bed by first placing mattress pad (if used). Fold lengthwise, ensuring crease is in center of bed. Likewise, unfold bottom sheet and place over mattress pad. Place hem of bottom sheet (if flat sheet is used) with rough edge down and just even with bottom edge of mattress. ☐ ☐ _____

i. Miter corners (if flat sheet) at head of bed. Continue to tuck in sheet along side toward front, keeping linens smooth. ☐ ☐ _____

j. Reach under patient to pull out protective draw sheet (if used), and smooth out over clean bottom sheet. Tuck in. Unfold linen draw sheet and place center fold along middle of bed, smooth out over protective draw sheet, and tuck in. Tuck in folded linens in center of bed so they are under patient's buttocks and torso. ☐ ☐ _____

k. Keep palms down as linens are tucked under mattress. ☐ ☐ _____

l. Raise side rail and assist patient to roll slowly toward you over folds of linen. Go to opposite side of bed and lower side rail. ☐ ☐ _____

m. Loosen edges of all soiled linens. Remove by folding into a bundle, and place in laundry bag ☐ ☐ _____

n. Spread clean linens, including protective draw sheet, out over mattress and smooth out wrinkles. Assist patient to supine position and position pillow for comfort. ☐ ☐ _____

o. Miter top corner of bottom sheet, pulling sheet taut. Tuck bottom sheet under mattress all the way to foot of bed. ☐ ☐ _____

p. Smooth out draw sheets. Pulling sheet taut, tuck in protective draw sheet and then tuck in linen draw sheet, first in center, then top, and bottom last. ☐ ☐ _____

q. Place top sheet over bath blanket that is over patient. Request patient to hold top sheet while you remove bath blanket. Place blanket in laundry bag. If blanket is used, place over sheet and place spread over blanket. Form cuff with top linens under patient's chin. ☐ ☐ _____

	S	U	Comments

r. Tuck in all linens at foot of bed, making modified miter corner. Raise side rail and make opposite side of bed. Remember to allow for toe pleat. Make toe pleat by placing fold either lengthwise down center of bed or across foot of bed. □ □ _____

s. Change pillowcase. Grasp closed end of pillowcase, turning case inside out over hand. Now grasp one end of pillow with your hand in the case and smooth out wrinkles, ensuring pillow corners fit into pillowcase corners. As pillow is removed from under patient, support neck muscles. Never hold pillow under your chin. □ □ _____

9. Unoccupied bed:

   a. Starting at head of bed, loosen linens all the way to foot. Go to opposite side of bed, loosen linens, roll all linens up in ball, and place in soiled laundry bag. Do not permit linens to come in contact with uniform. Do not shake or fan linens. Wash hands after handling soiled linens. Perform hand hygiene. □ □ _____

   b. If blanket and spread are to be reused, fold neatly and place over back of chair. Remove soiled pillowcase. □ □ _____

   c. Slide mattress to head of bed. □ □ _____

   d. If necessary, clean mattress with cloth moistened with antiseptic solution, and dry thoroughly. □ □ _____

   e. Begin to make bed standing on side where lines are placed. Unfold bottom sheet, placing fold lengthwise down center of bed. Be certain rough edge of hem lies down away from patient's heels and even with edge of mattress. Smooth out sheet over top edge of mattress and miter corners. Tuck remaining sheet under mattress all the way to foot. Keep linens smooth. □ □ _____

   f. Place draw sheet on bed so that center fold lies down middle of bed. If protective draw sheet is to be used, place it on first. Smooth out over mattress and tuck in. Keep palms down. □ □ _____

   g. Place top sheet over bed and smooth out. Place blanket over top sheet. Smooth out. Place spread over blanket and smooth out. Make cuff with top linens. □ □ _____

   h. Allow for toe pleat. Make modified mitered corner by not tucking tip of sheet under mattress. □ □ _____

213

	S	U	Comments

i. Move to opposite side of bed and complete making bed as described in steps 9e to 9h. Pull linens tight and keep taut as linens are tucked in.   ☐ ☐ _____

j. Put on clean pillowcase. Place pillow at head of bed and position for comfort. Place call light within easy reach and lower bed level.   ☐ ☐ _____

k. If patient is to return to bed, fan fold top linens down to foot of bed. Be sure cuff at top of linens is easily accessible to patient.   ☐ ☐ _____

10. Arrange personal items on bed table or bedside stand and place within patient's easy reach.   ☐ ☐ _____

11. Leave area neat and clean.   ☐ ☐ _____

12. Place all soiled linens in proper receptacle. Perform hand hygiene.   ☐ ☐ _____

13. Assist patient to bed and position for comfort.   ☐ ☐ _____

14. Documentation:

Bed making does not have to be recorded in most facilities.   ☐ ☐ _____

Record patient's vital signs, and signs and symptoms only if changes occur.   ☐ ☐ _____

15. Report any abnormal findings to nurse in charge.   ☐ ☐ _____

PROCEDURE 19-1

GIVING HAIR CARE

	S	U	Comments
1. Verify with the nurse the need for a shampoo.	☐	☐	_____
2. Introduce self.	☐	☐	_____
3. Identify patient.	☐	☐	_____
4. Explain procedure.	☐	☐	_____
5. Perform hand hygiene and don clean gloves according to agency policy and guidelines from the CDC and OSHA.	☐	☐	_____
6. Prepare patient.	☐	☐	_____
7. Close door or pull privacy curtain.			
8. Raise bed to a comfortable working height.	☐	☐	_____
9. Arrange supplies at bedside or, if patient is able to perform procedure, have supplies available in the bathroom and offer assistance as needed.	☐	☐	_____
10. Bed shampoo:	☐	☐	_____
a. Position patient close to one side of bed. Place shampoo board under patient's head and washbasin at end of spout. Ensure spout extends over edge of mattress.	☐	☐	_____
b. Position rolled-up bath towel under patient's neck. Certain conditions such as cervical neck injuries, open incisions, or tracheostomy place the patient at risk for injury, in which case, a modified position is used.	☐	☐	_____
c. Brush and comb patient's hair. If hair is matted with blood, hydrogen peroxide is effective as a cleansing agent.	☐	☐	_____
d. Obtain water in pitcher at about 110° F.	☐	☐	_____
e. If patient is able, instruct patient to hold washcloth over eyes. Completely wet hair and apply small amount of shampoo.	☐	☐	_____
f. Massage scalp with pads of fingertips, not nails. Shampoo hairline, back of neck(lift head slightly), and sides of hair.	☐	☐	_____

	S	U	Comments
g. Rinse thoroughly and apply more shampoo, repeating steps e and f. Rinse,and repeat rinsing until hair is free of shampoo.	☐	☐	_____
h. Wrap dry towel around patient's head. Dry patient's face, neck, and shoulders. Dry hair and scalp with second towel.	☐	☐	_____
i. Comb hair and dry with hair dryer as quickly as possible.	☐	☐	_____
j. Complete styling hair and position patient for comfort.	☐	☐	_____
k. Report abnormal findings (breaks in the skin or ulcerations) to nurse in charge.	☐	☐	_____

PROCEDURE 19-2

SHAVING THE PATIENT

	S	U	Comments
1. Verify with the nurse the need for a shave.	☐	☐	_____
2. Assemble supplies.			
3. Introduce self.	☐	☐	_____
4. Identify patient.	☐	☐	_____
5. Explain procedure.	☐	☐	_____
6. Perform hand hygiene and don clean gloves according to agency policy and guidelines from the CDC and OSHA.	☐	☐	_____
7. Prepare patient for intervention:			
a. Close door or pull privacy curtain.	☐	☐	_____
b. Raise bed to a comfortable working height.	☐	☐	_____
c. Arrange supplies at bedside or, if patient is able to perform procedure, have supplies available in the bathroom and offer assistance as needed.	☐	☐	_____
8. Shaving the patient:			
a. Assist patient to sitting position if patient is able.	☐	☐	_____
b. Observe face and neck for lesions, moles, or birthmarks.	☐	☐	_____
c. Use shaving cream or soap if an electric razor is not available.	☐	☐	_____
d. Shave in direction hair grows. Use short strokes. Start with upper face and lips, and then extend to neck. If patient is able, hyperextending his head is helpful to shave curved areas.	☐	☐	_____
e. Pull skin taut with nondominant hand above or below the area being shaved.	☐	☐	_____
f. Rinse razor after each stroke if using a disposable razor.	☐	☐	_____
g. Rinse and dry face.	☐	☐	_____
h. If patient desires, apply lotion or cologne.	☐	☐	_____
i. Dispose of blades in sharps container.	☐	☐	_____
j. Report abnormal findings (breaks in the skin or ulcerations) to nurse in charge.	☐	☐	_____

217

This page intentionally left blank

PROCEDURE 19-3

GIVING NAIL AND FOOT CARE

	S	U	Comments
1. Verify with the nurse the need for nail and foot care.	☐	☐	_____
2. Assemble supplies.	☐	☐	_____
3. Introduce self.	☐	☐	_____
4. Identify patient.	☐	☐	_____
5. Explain procedure.	☐	☐	_____
6. Verify with nurse any of the following:			
Contraindications to nail care	☐	☐	_____
Restrictions to positioning	☐	☐	_____
Condition of nails and feet; color and temperature of toes, feet, and fingers	☐	☐	_____
7. Perform hand hygiene and don clean gloves according to agency policy and guidelines from the CDC and OSHA.	☐	☐	_____
8. Prepare patient for intervention:			
a. Close door or pull privacy curtain.	☐	☐	_____
b. Raise bed to a comfortable working height.	☐	☐	_____
c. Arrange supplies at bedside or, if patient is able to perform procedure, have supplies available in the bathroom and offer assistance as needed.	☐	☐	_____
9. Hand and foot care:			
a. Position patient in chair. If possible, place disposable mat under patient's feet.	☐	☐	_____
b. Fill basin with warm water and test temperature. Place basin on disposable mat and assist patient to place feet into basin. Allow to soak 10 to 20 minutes. Rewarm water as necessary.	☐	☐	_____
c. Place overbed table in low position in front of patient. Fill emesis basin with warm water and test water temperature. Place basin on table, and place patient's fingers in basin. Allow fingernails to soak 10 to 20 minutes. Rewarm water as necessary.	☐	☐	_____

	S	U	Comments

d. Using orangewood stick, gently clean under fingernails. With clippers, trim nails straight across and even with tip of fingers. With emery board, shape fingernails. Push cuticles back gently with washcloth or orangewood stick. □ □ _____

e. Don gloves, and with washcloth scrub areas of feet that are calloused. □ □ _____

f. Trim and clean toenails following step d instructions. □ □ _____

g. Apply lotion or cream to hands and feet. Return patient to bed and position for comfort. Dry fingers and toes thoroughly to impede fungal growth and prevent maceration. Do not apply lotion between toes of patients with diabetes. □ □ _____

h. On completion of procedure, observe the nails and the surrounding tissue for condition of skin and any remaining rough edges. □ □ _____

i. If the patient's nails are extremely hard or if the patient is unable to perform personal nail care, have a podiatrist provide nail care. □ □ _____

j. Teach the patient with diabetes about appropriate foot care. The teaching plan includes inspecting the feet daily for breaks, wearing shoes at all times, wearing socks, drying feet completely, and noting any areas of numbness, tingling, or pain. □ □ _____

10. Dispose of gloves in proper receptacle. Clean and store supplies. Place soiled laundry in hamper. Perform hand hygiene. □ □ _____

11. Assess for patient's comfort, lower bed level, raise side rails, and place call button within easy reach. □ □ _____

12. Document:

Procedure □ □ _____

Pertinent observations □ □ _____

Most facilities have flow sheets for ADLs; know agency policy. □ □ _____

Report abnormal findings to nurse in charge. □ □ _____

PROCEDURE 19-4

DRESSING AND UNDRESSING THE PATIENT

	S	U	Comments

1. Verify with the nurse the need for changing the patient's clothes. ☐ ☐ _____

2. Assemble supplies. ☐ ☐ _____

3. Introduce self. ☐ ☐ _____

4. Identify patient. ☐ ☐ _____

5. Explain procedure. ☐ ☐ _____

6. Verify with nurse any of the following: any existing drainage tubes, dressings. ☐ ☐ _____

7. Be sure to pull the curtain. ☐ ☐ _____

8. If the patient is able to assist you with dressing, ask him/her to stand at the bedside. If patient is unable to provide any assistance, lower the bed rail and raise the bed to a height that is appropriate for good body mechanics. ☐ ☐ _____

Undressing the Patient

9. Untie the patient's gown from behind the neck and backside. If the patient is wearing street clothes, unfasten any snaps, buckles, or buttons. Take care to not drag the patient's skin across the bed linens as you reach to the back to untie the gown. You may need to have the patient roll to one side of the bed while you untie the gown. Have him/her roll to the other side to remove the gown from the second side. ☐ ☐ _____

10. Raise the patient's top piece of clothing to the shoulders, being sure to support the head if needed. Remove the strong arm from the sleeve of the garment first. Use the bath blanket to cover any areas which are revealed when removing the patient's top. ☐ ☐ _____

11. Remove the sleeve of the weak arm second. ☐ ☐ _____

12. Place the new gown on and tie in the back and around the neck. If the top garment is a shirt or sweater, gently place over the patient's head, being sure to not twist the head and neck. ☐ ☐ _____

221

	S	U	Comments

13. To remove the clothing from the lower part of the body, take any shoes off of the patient. Undo any buttons, unzip zippers, and unsnap any snaps. ☐ ☐ _____

14. If the person is lying in bed, ask him/her to raise the hips slightly off of the bed. ☐ ☐ _____

15. If the person is unable to lift the hips off the bed, turn the patient towards you and gently slide the pants down the strong side until it's below the hip and buttocks. Roll the person to the other side and do the same. Once the patient is supine again, lower the pants to the patient's feet. Use the bath blanket to cover the person's lower extremities while removing the pants. ☐ ☐ _____

16. Gently slide the pants down over the buttocks and down to the feet. ☐ ☐ _____

17. If the patient is able to stand, gently slide the pants down beneath the buttocks and hips to the ankles. Be careful to not allow the cuffs of the pants to get stuck around the foot as the person steps out of the pants. ☐ ☐ _____

Dressing the Patient

18. If the patient is lying supine in the bed, keep the bath blanket over top of the patient until he/she is completely dressed. ☐ ☐ _____

19. Be sure buttons, zippers, and snaps are undone or opened before trying to dress the patient. For tops that open in the back, slide the arm of the weak side into the sleeve opening. ☐ ☐ _____

20. Slide the arm of the strong side into the sleeve opening next. ☐ ☐ _____

21. If the patient is able to lift his/her head, pull the opening of the top over the patient's head and down over the chest. ☐ ☐ _____

22. Fasten the closure in the back. ☐ ☐ _____

23. For tops that open in the front, slide the sleeve of the top onto the arm that is on the weak side. ☐ ☐ _____

24. If the patient can raise his/her head and shoulders, bring the garment around the back to the other side. Then slide the sleeve on to the arm of the strong side. ☐ ☐ _____

	S	U	Comments
25. If the patient cannot raise his/her head or shoulders, then have the patient turn towards you and lie on his/her side.	☐	☐	_____
26. Take the top and tuck it underneath the patient.	☐	☐	_____
27. Turn the patient to the other side, with his/her back towards you.	☐	☐	_____
28. Pull the garment that was tucked underneath out and then turn the person back onto his/her back in a supine position.	☐	☐	_____
29. Take the clothing top and place it on the arm of the strong side.	☐	☐	_____
30. For pants or a skirt, slide the pants or skirt over the feet and onto the lower legs.	☐	☐	_____
31. Once the person lowers the hips to the bed, fasten any closures and button buttons,zip zippers, etc.	☐	☐	_____
32. If the patient can lift the hips, have him/her raise them slightly off the bed. Lift the pants or skirt up the legs and to the waist.	☐	☐	_____
33. If the patient is standing, have him/her lift one foot at a time and place the opening of the pants onto the foot and pull the pant leg upwards. Repeat for the second foot. Be sure to steady the patient by having him/her hold onto a bedrail or bathroom bar rail.	☐	☐	_____
34. Assist the patient with fastening any closures, buttons, zippers, etc.	☐	☐	_____
35. Put socks and shoes on the patient if he/she will be walking; if the patient will remain bed, place only socks on the feet.	☐	☐	_____
36. Always lower the bed back to the original position.	☐	☐	_____
37. Place the patient's call light within reach.	☐	☐	_____
38. Remove the privacy curtain.	☐	☐	_____

This page intentionally left blank

Student Name_____ Date_____

PROCEDURE 19-5

CHANGING THE GOWN OF A PATIENT WITH AN IV LINE

	S	U	Comments
1. Verify with the nurse the need for changing the gown.	☐	☐	_____
2. Assemble supplies.	☐	☐	_____
3. Introduce self.	☐	☐	_____
4. Identify patient.	☐	☐	_____
5. Explain procedure.	☐	☐	_____
6. Raise the patient's bed to a level that is appropriate for you.	☐	☐	_____
7. Cover the patient with a bath blanket.	☐	☐	_____
8. Untie the patient's gown from behind the neck.	☐	☐	_____
9. Slide the gown down the arm that does not have the IV.	☐	☐	_____
10. Take the sleeve of the arm with the IV and pull it gently over the IV site and tubing, taking care to not catch or pull on the IV site.	☐	☐	_____
11. Holding the material of the gown with one hand, remove the patient's hand from the sleeve of the gown with the other hand.	☐	☐	_____
12. Take the bag of the IV, keeping it at as close to the same height as it was on the pole as possible, and pull it through the sleeve of the gown. If the IV bag is on a pump or electronic infusion device, the nurse will need to assist the PCT, to ensure the roller clamp is slowed or clamped before removing to prevent an infusion of a large volume of solution or medication.	☐	☐	_____
13. The clean gown is passed through the opening of the arm sleeve in the gown from the opening up towards the shoulder of the gown and then replaced on the pole.	☐	☐	_____

This page intentionally left blank

PROCEDURE 21-1

ASSISTING PATIENTS WITH EATING

	S	U	Comments
1. Complete or delay care that will interfere with eating.	☐	☐	_____
2. Provide a period of rest or quiet before meals.	☐	☐	_____
3. Offer the patient a bedpan or urinal before mealtime.	☐	☐	_____
4. Provide the patient with an opportunity for handwashing, and offer mouth care before the meal.	☐	☐	_____
5. Remove soiled articles or clutter from room.	☐	☐	_____
6. Make the patient comfortable for eating; give pain medication at least 30 minutes prior to a meal.	☐	☐	_____
7. Raise the head of the bed to a sitting position.	☐	☐	_____
8. Cover the patient's upper chest with a napkin or some form of clothing protector.	☐	☐	_____
9. Sit beside the patient to assist with feeding.	☐	☐	_____
10. Encourage patients to feed themselves as much as possible.	☐	☐	_____
11. Provide a flexible straw for patients who are unable to use a cup or glass.	☐	☐	_____
12. Serve manageable amounts of food in each bite.	☐	☐	_____
13. For a patient who has had a stroke, direct the food toward the side of the mouth not affected by the stroke.	☐	☐	_____
14. Serve food in the order of the patient's preference.	☐	☐	_____
15. Give the patient time to chew and swallow food.	☐	☐	_____
16. Modify utensils and texture of food if the patient has to remain flat while eating. Use a training cup or a large syringe with flexible rubber tube. Purée or grind foods.	☐	☐	_____
17. During the feeding, do not leave the patient until he or she has finished eating. Do not interrupt the meal.	☐	☐	_____
18. Carry on pleasant conversation with patient during the meal.	☐	☐	_____
19. Remove the tray from the patient's room as soon as the meal is completed.	☐	☐	_____

This page intentionally left blank

PROCEDURE 21-2

MEASURING INTAKE AND OUTPUT

	S	U	Comments
1. Identify patient.	☐	☐	_____
2. Explain procedure.	☐	☐	_____
3. Instruct patient to inform staff of all oral intake. Provide a marked intake and output (I&O) container.	☐	☐	_____
4. Instruct patient not to empty any output collection receptacles and to notify the nurse after elimination.	☐	☐	_____
5. Alert all staff and remind patient of need to measure I&O.	☐	☐	_____
6. Measure and record all fluids taken orally, gastric tube feedings, and all fluids administered parenterally.	☐	☐	_____
7. Wash hands and don gloves.	☐	☐	_____
8. Measure and record output in Foley drainage system, diarrhea stools, nasogastric suction, emesis, ileostomy, and surgical wound receptacles such as Davol, Jackson-Pratt, and Hemovac drains. Measure and record output from chest tube drainage in water-seal container by marking with felt-tip pen.	☐	☐	_____
9. Remove gloves and wash hands.	☐	☐	_____
10. Compute I&O, and document it on patient's record.	☐	☐	_____

This page intentionally left blank

PROCEDURE 21-3

DISCONTINUING A PERIPHERAL IV SITE

	S	U	Comments
1. Assemble equipment.	☐	☐	_____
2. Perform hand hygiene.	☐	☐	_____
3. Explain to the patient what you are going to do.	☐	☐	_____
4. Remove any overlying tape. Then remove transparent membrane dressing by picking up one corner and pulling the side laterally while holding catheter hub. Repeat for other side.	☐	☐	_____
a. Alternative is to remove gauze dressing and tape from site one layer at a time by pulling toward the insertion site. Tape securing catheter to skin should be left intact.	☐	☐	_____
5. Site evaluation:	☐	☐	_____
a. Review health care provider's orders or verify with the nurse for discontinuation of IV therapy.	☐	☐	_____
b. Determine patient's understanding of the need for removal of peripheral IV catheter.	☐	☐	_____
6. Explain procedure to patient.	☐	☐	_____
7. Turn IV tubing roller clamp to "off" position. Remove tape securing tubing.	☐	☐	_____
8. Remove IV site dressing and tape while stabilizing catheter.	☐	☐	_____
9. With dry gauze held over site, apply light pressure and withdraw the catheter, using a slow steady movement, keeping the hub parallel to the skin.	☐	☐	_____
10. Apply pressure to the site for 2 to 3 minutes, using a dry, sterile gauze pad. Secure the tape over the gauze snugly.	☐	☐	_____
11. Inspect the catheter for intactness, noting tip integrity and length.	☐	☐	_____
12. Discard used supplies.	☐	☐	_____
13. Remove and discard gloves, and performh and hygiene.	☐	☐	_____
14. Instruct patient to report any erythema, pain, drainage, or edema that occurs after catheter removal.	☐	☐	_____

231

	S	U	Comments

15. Document and record the following:

    a. Time peripheral IV infusion was discontinued ☐ ☐ _____

    b. Condition of site ☐ ☐ _____

    c. Gauge and length of catheter ☐ ☐ _____

    d. Whether catheter is intact ☐ ☐ _____

PROCEDURE 22-1

POSITIONING THE BEDPAN

	S	U	Comments
1. Refer to medical record, care plan, or Kardex.	☐	☐	_____
2. Assess patient's needs.	☐	☐	_____
3. Assemble supplies according to patient's needs.	☐	☐	_____
4. Introduce self.	☐	☐	_____
5. Identify patient.	☐	☐	_____
6. Explain procedure.	☐	☐	_____
7. Prepare patient:	☐	☐	_____
a. Close door or pull privacy curtain.	☐	☐	_____
b. Arrange supplies close to the bedside.	☐	☐	_____
c. Place protective pad under patient's buttocks, if necessary.	☐	☐	_____
8. Perform hand hygiene and don clean gloves according to agency policy and guidelines from the CDC and OSHA.	☐	☐	_____
9. When patient is able to assist self onto bedpan, position patient in supine position with knees flexed and bottom of feet flat on bed surface. As patient raises hips, support patient's lower back with arm and positions bedpan under patient. When patient has finished with elimination, remove bedpan in same manner.	☐	☐	_____
10. For patient unable to assist self on bedpan:			
a. Turn patient away from yourself toward opposite side rail, moving linens out of way.	☐	☐	_____
b. Fit bedpan to patient's buttocks.	☐	☐	_____
c. Assist patient to turn over onto bedpan while securing bedpan.	☐	☐	_____
d. Raise head of bed 30 degrees.	☐	☐	_____
e. Place toilet tissue and call light within easy reach.	☐	☐	_____
11. If the male patient is unable to place a urinal for himself, you need to assist him.			
a. Request that the patient abduct his legs aslight distance.	☐	☐	_____

	S	U	Comments

b. Holding the urinal by the handle and directing the urinal at an angle, place the urinal between the patient's legs, making certain the long flat side, which is opposite the handle of the urinal, is resting on the bed.   ☐ ☐ _____

c. Gently raising the penis, place it fully within the urinal.   ☐ ☐ _____

d. Provide for privacy while the patient urinates.   ☐ ☐ _____

e. Once he signals he is finished, provide toilet paper to dry the tip of the penis.   ☐ ☐ _____

f. Rinse the urinal with water before returning to its storage area (usually in the bottom cabinet of the bedside cabinet).   ☐ ☐ _____

12. For those patients who can be out of bed but are unable to ambulate far, the bedside commode can be used. Some are equipped with wheels, which allow the patient to be moved to the bathroom.   ☐ ☐ _____

13. When transferring a patient to the commode, assist the patient in the same manner as if assisting to a chair.   ☐ ☐ _____

14. Provide a means for the patient to wash hands; either assisting to the sink or providing hand washing while patient is in the bed.   ☐ ☐ _____

15. Remove your gloves and practice hand hygiene.   ☐ ☐ _____

16. Provide for the patient's comfort by returning the bed to its original position.   ☐ ☐ _____

17. Place the call light within reach.   ☐ ☐ _____

18. Lower the bed to its original position.   ☐ ☐ _____

19. Document the procedure, noting any abnormal observations.   ☐ ☐ _____

20. Document according to agency policy: ☐ ☐ _____

     Amount   ☐ ☐ _____

     Color   ☐ ☐ _____

     Consistency   ☐ ☐ _____

     Abnormal findings such as blood, unusual odor, or color   ☐ ☐ _____

21. Report unusual findings.   ☐ ☐ _____

PROCEDURE 22-2

USING A BLADDER SCANNER TO MEASURE POSTVOID RESIDUAL

	S	U	Comments
1. Refer to medical record, care plan, or Kardex.	☐	☐	_____
2. Assess patient's needs.	☐	☐	_____
3. Assemble supplies according to patient's needs.	☐	☐	_____
4. Introduce self.	☐	☐	_____
5. Identify patient.	☐	☐	_____
6. Explain procedure.	☐	☐	_____
7. Prepare patient:			
a. Close door or pull privacy curtain.	☐	☐	_____
b. Arrange supplies close to the bedside.	☐	☐	_____
c. Place protective pad under patient's buttocks, if necessary.	☐	☐	_____
8. Perform hand hygiene and don clean gloves according to agency policy and guidelines from the CDC and OSHA.	☐	☐	_____
9. Pull back sheet to expose patient's lower abdomen.	☐	☐	_____
10. Turn on scanner per manufacturer guidelines. Set gender designation per manufacturer guidelines. Women who have had a hysterectomy should be designated as male.	☐	☐	_____
11. Wipe scanner head with alcohol pad or other cleaner and allow to air dry.	☐	☐	_____
12. Palpate the patient's pubic bone. Apply a generous amount of ultrasound gel to the midline of the abdomen 2.5 to 4 cm above the symphysis pubis.	☐	☐	_____
13. Place scanner head on gel.	☐	☐	_____
14. Apply light pressure, keep scanner head steady, and point it slightly downward toward bladder. Press and release the scan button.	☐	☐	_____
15. Verify accurate aim. Complete scan and print image if needed.	☐	☐	_____

	S	U	Comments
16. Remove ultrasound gel from patient's abdomen with paper towel or moist cloth.	☐	☐	_____
17. Remove ultrasound gel from scanner head and wipe with alcohol pad or other cleaner; allow to air-dry.	☐	☐	_____
18. Help patient to a comfortable position. Raise side rails as appropriate, or lower bed to lowest position.	☐	☐	_____
19. Be sure the call light is within the patient's reach.	☐	☐	_____
20. Remove and dispose of gloves and perform hand hygiene.	☐	☐	_____
21. Document the results of the PVR and patient tolerance of the procedure on the patient's chart.	☐	☐	_____

PROCEDURE 22-3

CATHETERIZATION: MALE AND FEMALE PATIENTS

	S	U	Comments
1. Refer to medical record, care plan, or Kardex.	☐	☐	_____
2. Assess patient's needs.	☐	☐	_____
3. Assemble supplies according to patient's needs.	☐	☐	_____
4. Introduce self.	☐	☐	_____
5. Identify patient.	☐	☐	_____
6. Explain procedure.	☐	☐	_____
7. Prepare patient.	☐	☐	_____
8. Close door or pull privacy curtain.	☐	☐	_____
9. Arrange supplies close to the bedside.	☐	☐	_____
10. Place protective pad under patient's buttocks, if necessary.	☐	☐	_____
11. Perform hand hygiene and don clean gloves according to agency policy and guidelines from the CDC and OSHA.	☐	☐	_____
12. Determine the following:	☐	☐	_____
a. When patient last voided	☐	☐	_____
b. Patient's level of awareness	☐	☐	_____
c. Mobility and physical limitation of patient	☐	☐	_____
d. Patient's sex and age	☐	☐	_____
e. Whether patient's bladder is distended	☐	☐	_____
f. Presence of any pathologic conditions that are likely to impair passage of catheter	☐	☐	_____
g. Allergies (to antiseptic [iodine], tape, rubber, and lubricant)	☐	☐	_____
h. Patient's knowledge of the purpose of catheterization	☐	☐	_____
13. Arrange for extra assistive personnel to assist if needed.	☐	☐	_____
14. Position patient.	☐	☐	_____

	S	U	Comments

a. Male patient: Supine position with thighs slightly abducted.

b. Female patient: Supine position with knees flexed and knees about 2 feet apart.

15. Drape patient with bath blanket, covering upper body and shaping over both knees and legs but leaving genital area exposed.

16. Place waterproof absorbent pad under patient's buttocks.

17. Arrange supplies and equipment on bedside table. Provide a good light.

18. Don clean gloves, and wash perineal area with mild soap and warm water.

19. Remove disposable gloves, and place them in proper receptacle.

20. Facing patient, stand on left side of bed if right-handed (on right side if left-handed).

21. Open packaging with the use of sterile technique. Don sterile gloves.

22. If indwelling catheter is used, test balloon by injecting normal saline or sterile water into balloon lumen until balloon is inflated; then aspirate saline or sterile water out of balloon.

23. Add antiseptic to cotton balls; open lubricant container. Lubricate catheter approximately1.5 to 2 inches (3.5 to 5 cm) for female patient and approximately 6 to 7 inches (15 to 18 cm)for male patient.

24. Wrap edges of sterile drape around gloved hands, and request patient to raise hips; then slide drape under patient's buttocks.

25. Cleanse perineal area with forceps to hold cotton balls soaked in antiseptic solution.

a. Male: If male patient is not circumcised, retract foreskin with nondominant hand. Be certain to replace foreskin when procedure has been completed. If erection occurs,discontinue procedure momentarily. This is normal but often embarrassing to patient. React in a professional manner. Grasp penis at shaft below glans with nondominant hand; continue to hold throughout insertion of catheter. The nondominant hand is no longer sterile and must not come in contact with sterile supplies.

	S	U	Comments

(1) With other hand, use forceps to pick up cotton balls soaked in antiseptic solution. Cleanse meatus by beginning at top of penis and moving in a circular motion down and around meatus one time. Discard cotton ball in appropriate receptacle. ☐ ☐ _____

(2) Repeat cleansing two more times with sterile cotton balls each time. ☐ ☐ _____

b. Female:

(1) Spread labia minora with thumb and index finger of nondominant hand to expose meatus; continue to hold throughout insertion of catheter. The nondominant hand is no longer sterile and must not come in contact with sterile supplies. ☐ ☐ _____

(2) With other hand, use forceps to pick up cotton balls soaked in antiseptic solution. ☐ ☐ _____

(3) Cleanse area from clitoris toward anus. Use a different sterile cotton ball each time: first to the right of the meatus, then to the left of the meatus, then down the center over meatus. ☐ ☐ _____

26. Pick up catheter with dominant sterile-gloved hand near the tip; hold remaining part of catheter coiled in hands; place distal end in basin. ☐ ☐ _____

27. Insert catheter gently, about 6 to 7 inches (15 to 18 cm) for male patient or 2 to 4 inches (5 to 10 cm) for female patient. Once urine flow is established, insert catheter 1.5 inches (3.5 cm) farther. *(Advancement of catheter ensures correct bladder placement.)* Inflate balloon with 10 mL of sterile water. Gently pull back on catheter until resistance is felt as balloon rests at orifice of urethra. In a female patient, if no urine returns in a few minutes, observe whether catheter has been inserted by mistake into vagina. If so, leave catheter in place as landmark indicating where not to insert, and insert another sterile catheter. ☐ ☐ _____

a. Indwelling catheter:

(1) Inflate balloon with required amount of normal saline or sterile water. ☐ ☐ _____

(2) Pull gently to feel resistance. ☐ ☐ _____

(3) Collect urine specimen, if needed, by placing open lumen end of catheter into specimen container. ☐ ☐ _____

(4) Attach open lumen of catheter to collecting tube of drainage system, holding drainage bag below bladder level. ☐ ☐ _____

	S	U	Comments
(5) Attach collection bag to a stationary part on the side of bed.	☐	☐	_____
(6) Secure catheter to patient.	☐	☐	_____
(a) Male patient: Tape catheter to inner aspect of thigh or up over pubis, or apply leg strap (depends on health care provider's order); allow slack for body movement.	☐	☐	_____
(b) Female patient: Tape catheter to inner thigh or apply leg strap; allow slack for body movement.	☐	☐	_____
(7) Clip drainage tubing to bed linen; allow slack for body movement.	☐	☐	_____
b. Straight catheter:			
(1) Once urine flow is established, hold open lumen of catheter over basin.	☐	☐	_____
(2) Empty bladder (approximately 700 to 1000 mL). Refer to facility policy to determine whether urine should be allowed to continue draining.	☐	☐	_____
(3) Collect urine specimen, if needed, by placing open lumen end of catheter into specimen container.	☐	☐	_____
(4) Withdraw catheter slowly.	☐	☐	_____
28. Wash and dry perineal area.	☐	☐	_____
29. Label urine specimen with patient's name, date, health care provider's name, and other information as required by facility. Ensure urine is transported to laboratory.	☐	☐	_____
30. Check flow of urine and drainage tubing.	☐	☐	_____
31. Remove your gloves and practice hand hygiene.	☐	☐	_____
32. Provide for the patient's comfort by returning the bed to its original position.	☐	☐	_____
33. Place the call light within reach.	☐	☐	_____
34. Lower the bed to its original position.	☐	☐	_____
35. Document the procedure, noting any abnormal observations.	☐	☐	_____
Date and time of procedure	☐	☐	_____

	S	U	Comments
Type and size of catheter	☐	☐	_____
Amount of solution used to inflate balloon	☐	☐	_____
Characteristics of urine	☐	☐	_____
Amount of urine	☐	☐	_____
Color of urine and consistency of urine (note particles in urine)	☐	☐	_____
Specimen collected	☐	☐	_____
Patient's response to procedure (any resistance met)	☐	☐	_____
36. Report any unusual findings immediately.	☐	☐	_____
No urine output	☐	☐	_____
Bladder discomfort despite catheter patency	☐	☐	_____
Leakage of urine from catheter	☐	☐	_____
Inability to insert catheter	☐	☐	_____

This page intentionally left blank

PROCEDURE 22-4

PERFORMING ROUTINE CATHETER CARE

	S	U	Comments
1. Refer to medical record, care plan, or Kardex.	☐	☐	_____
2. Assess patient's needs.	☐	☐	_____
3. Assemble supplies according to patient's needs.	☐	☐	_____
4. Introduce self.	☐	☐	_____
5. Identify patient.	☐	☐	_____
6. Explain procedure.	☐	☐	_____
7. Prepare patient.			
Close door or pull privacy curtain.	☐	☐	_____
Arrange supplies close to the bedside.	☐	☐	_____
Place protective pad under patient's buttocks, if necessary.	☐	☐	_____
8. Perform hand hygiene and don clean gloves according to agency policy and guidelines from the CDC and OSHA.	☐	☐	_____
9. Assemble equipment.	☐	☐	_____
10. Evaluate patient for the following:			
a. Length of time catheter has been in place	☐	☐	_____
b. Encrustations or discharge around urethral meatus	☐	☐	_____
c. Complaints of pain and for allergies to antiseptic ointment	☐	☐	_____
d. Patient's temperature	☐	☐	_____
e. Patient's intake	☐	☐	_____
11. Position patient.			
a. Male: supine position in bed with thighs slightly abducted.	☐	☐	_____
b. Female: supine position in bed with knees flexed and knees about 2 feet apart.	☐	☐	_____
12. Place waterproof disposable pad under patient's buttocks.	☐	☐	_____
13. Drape patient with bath blanket, exposing only perineal area.	☐	☐	_____

	S	U	Comments

14. If sterile catheter care kit is to be used: ☐ ☐ _____

   a. Open supplies with sterile technique, and arrange them on bedside table. ☐ ☐ _____

   b. Don sterile gloves. ☐ ☐ _____

   c. Place cotton balls in sterile basin near the nurse, and saturate with antiseptic solution. ☐ ☐ _____

   d. With one hand, expose urethral meatus: ☐ ☐ _____

      (1) Male: Retract foreskin if it is present, then hold penis erect; hold position. ☐ ☐ _____

      (2) Female: Gently retract labia minora away from urinary meatus and hold in position. ☐ ☐ _____

   e. Wash the area at the meatus and around catheter with cotton balls soaked in antiseptic solution. ☐ ☐ _____

      (1) Male: ☐ ☐ _____

         (a) With one cotton ball, cleanse around meatus and catheter in a circular motion, starting at top of penis. ☐ ☐ _____

         (b) Repeat twice more, using different cotton balls each time. ☐ ☐ _____

      (2) Female:

         (a) With one cotton ball, swab to one side of labia minora from anterior to posterior. ☐ ☐ _____

         (b) Repeat with second cotton ball on opposite side. ☐ ☐ _____

         (c) Repeat with third cotton ball down middle over meatus and around catheter; do not bring cotton ball back up once descent has begun. ☐ ☐ _____

   f. Discard soiled cotton balls in other basin in kit. ☐ ☐ _____

   g. With forceps, pick up cotton ball soaked in antiseptic solution or use mild soap and water, and cleanse around catheter from urethral opening to approximately 4 inches(10 cm) of the catheter from the urethral opening. ☐ ☐ _____

15. If a collection of sterile supplies is to be used: ☐ ☐ _____

   a. Open separate sterile packages, observing sterile technique. ☐ ☐ _____

   b. Don clean gloves. ☐ ☐ _____

	S	U	Comments
c. Arrange small plastic bag for used, contaminated supplies.	☐	☐	_____
d. Cleanse the perineal area with mild soap and warm water. Pat dry.	☐	☐	_____
(1) Male: Retract foreskin if it is present; then hold the penis erect.	☐	☐	_____
(2) Female: Gently retract labia away from urinary meatus.	☐	☐	_____
e. Release labia of female patient; replace foreskin of male patient after cleaning.	☐	☐	_____
16. Observe meatus, catheter, and surrounding tissue to determine normal or abnormal condition. Note presence or absence of inflammation, edema, malodorous exudate, color of tissue, or burning sensation.	☐	☐	_____
17. Dispose of equipment and linens, according to Standard Precautions and facility policy; remove gloves and dispose of them in proper receptacle. Perform hand hygiene.	☐	☐	_____
18. Tape the catheter to thigh or use a catheter strap.	☐	☐	_____
19. Observe flow of urine through drainage tubing; note the accumulation of urine in the collecting receptacle. If the drainage tubing becomes cloudy or stained, change the tubing to aid accurate observations of urine. Emptyd rainage receptacle at least every 8 hours or as necessary to prevent backup of urinein to the tubing or bladder.	☐	☐	_____
20. Remove your gloves and practice hand hygiene.	☐	☐	_____
21. Provide for the patient's comfort by returning the bed to its original position.	☐	☐	_____
22. Place their call light within reach.	☐	☐	_____
23. Lower the bed to its original position.	☐	☐	_____
24. Document the procedure, noting any abnormal observations.	☐	☐	_____
25. Document the following:			
Date and time	☐	☐	_____
Procedure	☐	☐	_____
Assessment of urinary meatus	☐	☐	_____

	S	U	Comments
Character of urine	☐	☐	_____
Patient's response	☐	☐	_____
Patient teaching	☐	☐	_____
Report any unusual findings immediately.	☐	☐	_____

PROCEDURE 22-5

CHANGING A LEG BAG TO A DRAINAGE BAG AND EMPTYING A DRAINAGE BAG

	S	U	Comments
1. Refer to medical record, care plan, or Kardex.	☐	☐	_____
2. Assess patient's needs.	☐	☐	_____
3. Assemble supplies according to patient's needs.	☐	☐	_____
4. Introduce self.	☐	☐	_____
5. Identify patient.	☐	☐	_____
6. Explain procedure.	☐	☐	_____
7. Prepare patient.	☐	☐	_____
8. Close door or pull privacy curtain.	☐	☐	_____
9. Arrange supplies close to the bedside.	☐	☐	_____
10. Place protective on bed under patient's buttocks, if necessary.	☐	☐	_____
11. Perform hand hygiene and don clean gloves according to agency policy and guidelines from the CDC and OSHA.	☐	☐	_____
12. Assemble equipment.	☐	☐	_____
13. If able, have the person to sit on the edge of the bed.	☐	☐	_____
14. Don clean gloves, and gain access to the catheter and leg bag.	☐	☐	_____
15. Clamp the catheter using the clamp on the leg bag; urine below the clamp will continue to drain into the leg bag.	☐	☐	_____
16. Have the patient lie down on the bed in a supine position; cover him/her with the bath blanket (provides for privacy and warmth).	☐	☐	_____
17. Raise the bed to a height that promotes good body mechanics.	☐	☐	_____
18. Using the bedside table to organize your supplies, place a towel across the surface.	☐	☐	_____
19. Open the antiseptic wipes, sterile cap and plug, as well as the package with the drainage bag and tubing; do not touch the sterile cap or plug. These should be on the bedside table.	☐	☐	_____

247

	S	U	Comments

20. Attach the drainage bag to the bed frame. ☐ ☐ _____

21. Disconnect the catheter from the drainage tubing, taking great care to not touch the tip or opening of either. ☐ ☐ _____

22. Pick up the sterile plug by the package and not the exposed tip, and insert it into the catheter end. ☐ ☐ _____

23. Attach the sterile cap onto the end of the leg bag drainage tube. ☐ ☐ _____

24. Remove caps from the tubing of the new drainage bag, and the sterile plug, and connect the two by inserting one into the other. ☐ ☐ _____

25. Release the clamp on the catheter that is currently clamped; urine should begin to flow through the tubing. ☐ ☐ _____

26. Discard of the leg bag once you have drained and measured the urine.

   a. To empty the urinary drainage bag, open the clamp on the drain. ☐ ☐ _____

   b. Let all urine drain from the bag into a graduated cylinder. ☐ ☐ _____

   c. Reclamp the drain so that no remaining urine leaks onto the floor. ☐ ☐ _____

   d. Measure the amount of urine obtained in the graduated cylinder. ☐ ☐ _____

   e. Take the graduated cylinder to the bathroom to dispose of the urine in the toilet. ☐ ☐ _____

   f. Rinse the graduated cylinder with clean water. ☐ ☐ _____

   g. Return it to its storage location (usually located in the bathroom). ☐ ☐ _____

27. Remove the bath blanket and return the patient's covers or gown. ☐ ☐ _____

28. Take the bedpan and other disposable supplies to the bathroom. ☐ ☐ _____

29. Dispose of any urine in the toilet once it has been accounted for. ☐ ☐ _____

30. Dispose of any disposable supplies in the trashcan. ☐ ☐ _____

31. Rinse the bedpan and return to its location in the lower portion of the bedside cabinet. ☐ ☐ _____

	S	U	Comments
32. Remove your gloves and practice hand hygiene.	☐	☐	_____
33. Provide for the patient's comfort by returning the bed to its original position.	☐	☐	_____
34. Place the call light within reach.	☐	☐	_____
35. Lower the bed to its original position.	☐	☐	_____
36. Document the procedure, noting any abnormal observations.	☐	☐	_____

This page intentionally left blank

PROCEDURE 22-6

REMOVING AN INDWELLING CATHETER

	S	U	Comments
1. Refer to medical record, care plan, or Kardex.	☐	☐	_____
2. Assemble supplies according to patient's needs.	☐	☐	_____
3. Introduce self.	☐	☐	_____
4. Identify patient.	☐	☐	_____
5. Explain procedure.	☐	☐	_____
6. Prepare patient.	☐	☐	_____
7. Close door or pull privacy curtain.	☐	☐	_____
8. Arrange supplies close to the bedside.	☐	☐	_____
9. Place protective pad under patient's buttocks, if necessary.	☐	☐	_____
10. Perform hand hygiene and don clean gloves according to agency policy and guidelines from the CDC and OSHA.	☐	☐	_____
11. Assemble equipment:	☐	☐	_____
10-mL syringe or larger (depending on volume of fluid used to inflate balloon) without a needle	☐	☐	_____
12. Determine the following:	☐	☐	_____
a. Length of time catheter has been in place	☐	☐	_____
b. Patient's knowledge of procedure and what to expect	☐	☐	_____
13. Provide privacy. Position the patient supine, and place a waterproof pad under the patient's buttocks. Female patients need to abduct their legs with the drape between their thighs. For male patients, it is acceptable for drape to lie on the thighs.	☐	☐	_____
14. Insert hub of syringe into inflation valve (balloon port), and aspirate until tubing collapses or resistance is felt.	☐	☐	_____
15. Remove catheter steadily and smoothly (in female patients, the catheter is in about 2 to 3 inches [5 to 7.5 cm] and in male patients, about 6 to 7 inches [15 to 18 cm]). Catheter usually slides out very easily. Do not use force. If any resistance is noted, repeat step 5 to remove remaining water.	☐	☐	_____

251

Procedures Checklists

	S	U	Comments

16. Wrap catheter in waterproof pad. Unhook collection bag and drainage tubing from the bed. ☐ ☐ _____

17. Measure urine, and empty drainage bag. ☐ ☐ _____

18. Record output. ☐ ☐ _____

19. Cleanse the perineum with soap and warm water, and dry area thoroughly. ☐ ☐ _____

20. Explain the following to patient, as directed by the nurse:

   a. It is important to have a fluid intake of 1.5 to 2 L/day unless contraindicated. ☐ ☐ _____

   b. The patient must void within 8 hours, and each voiding should be measured. Some facilities and health care providers determine how much the patient should void to verify adequate emptying of the urinary bladder. ☐ ☐ _____

   c. Mild burning sensation or discomfort with first voiding is anticipated. Instruct patient to notify the nurse if it does not subside with subsequent voidings. ☐ ☐ _____

   d. Signs of urinary tract infection are urinary urgency, burning sensation, urinary frequency, excretion of only small amount, and continued pain or discomfort. These symptoms may develop 2 to 3 days after removal of catheter. ☐ ☐ _____

21. Place the urine measuring device on the toilet seat. ☐ ☐ _____

22. Document and report the following: ☐ ☐ _____

   Date and time of catheter removal ☐ ☐ _____

   Time, amount, and characteristics of first voiding after catheter removal ☐ ☐ _____

   Complete input and output record ☐ ☐ _____

PROCEDURE 23-1

ADMINISTERING AN ENEMA

	S	U	Comments
1. Check the health care provider's order.	☐	☐	_____
2. Introduce yourself to the patient; include your name and title or role.	☐	☐	_____
3. Identify the patient by checking his or her identification bracelet and requesting that the patient state his or her name or birth date, or both.	☐	☐	_____
4. Explain the procedure and the reason it is to be done in terms that the patient is able to understand. Advise the patient of any unpleasantness that may be involved with the procedure. Give the patient time to ask questions.	☐	☐	_____
5. Determine need for and provide patient education before and during procedure.	☐	☐	_____
6. Evaluate the patient.	☐	☐	_____
7. Perform hand hygiene and don clean gloves according to agency policy and guidelines from the Centers for Disease Control and Prevention (CDC) and the Occupational Safety and Health Administration (OSHA).	☐	☐	_____
8. Assemble equipment, and complete necessary charges.	☐	☐	_____
9. Prepare the patient for the procedure:			
a. Close the door or pull the privacy curtain around the patient's bed.	☐	☐	_____
b. Raise the bed to a comfortable working height, and lower the side rail on the side nearest the patient care technician.	☐	☐	_____
c. Position and drape the patient as necessary.	☐	☐	_____
10. Assemble equipment.	☐	☐	_____
11. Determine the following:			
a. Most recent bowel movement	☐	☐	_____
b. Presence or absence of bowel sounds	☐	☐	_____
c. Ability to control rectal sphincter	☐	☐	_____
d. Presence or absence of hemorrhoids	☐	☐	_____

253

	S	U	Comments

e. Presence of abdominal pain ☐ ☐ _____

f. Patient's level of understanding and previous experience with enemas ☐ ☐ _____

12. Prepare solution. There are several types of enema solution. Cleansing enemas include tap water, normal saline, low-volume hypertonic solutions, and soapsuds solution. ☐ ☐ _____

13. Arrange equipment at patient's bedside. ☐ ☐ _____

14. Assist patient to the Sims' position. When an enema is given to a patient who is unable to contract the external sphincter, position the patient on the bedpan. Avoid giving the enema with the patient sitting on the toilet; it is possible for the inserted rectal tubing to abrade the rectal wall, and the enema solution is forced upward, which makes the enema less effective. ☐ ☐ _____

15. Place waterproof pad under patient. ☐ ☐ _____

16. Place bath blanket over patient and fan fold linen to foot of bed; adjust patient's gown to keep it from being soiled while it still provides privacy. ☐ ☐ _____

17. Clamp tubing; fill container with correctly warmed solution (usually 750 to 1000 mL at105° F [41° C]) and any additives ordered. Administer a child's enema using appropriate equipment at 100° F to avoid burning rectal tissue; read disposable package for instructions. Release clamp, allowing solution to flow through tubing to remove any air from the tubing; reclamp. Suggested maximal volumes are as follows: ☐ ☐ _____

• Infant: 150 to 250 mL ☐ ☐ _____

• Toddler: 250 to 500 mL ☐ ☐ _____

• School-age child: 500 mL ☐ ☐ _____

• Adolescent: 500 to 700 mL ☐ ☐ _____

• Adult: 750 to 1000 mL ☐ ☐ _____

a. For commercially prepared enema: ☐ ☐ _____

(1) Remove cover from tip of enema (tip is prelubricated, but add lubricant if needed); insert entire tip into anus. ☐ ☐ _____

	S	U	Comments

(2) Squeeze container until it is empty. Usually a small amount of solution will remain in container. Most containers hold about 250 mL. Continue to squeeze the container to prevent siphoning solution back into the container. ☐ ☐ _____

(3) Encourage patient to retain solution at least 5 minutes. ☐ ☐ _____

  b. For standard enema:

(1) Lubricate 4 inches (10 cm) at end of tubing; spread patient's buttocks to expose anus; while rotating tube, gently insert it 3 to 4 inches (7 to 10 cm). Instruct patient to breathe out slowly through mouth. ☐ ☐ _____

(2) Elevate container 12 to 18 inches (30 to 45 cm) above level of anus. ☐ ☐ _____

(3) Release clamp, and allow solution to flow slowly. Usually solution will flow for 5 to 10 minutes. ☐ ☐ _____

(4) Lower container or clamp tubing if patient complains of cramping; encourage slow, deep breathing. Do not remove tubing tip. If severe cramping, bleeding, or sudden severe abdominal pain occurs and is unrelieved by temporarily stopping or slowing flow of solution, stop enema and notify health care provider. ☐ ☐ _____

(5) Clamp and remove tube when all of the solution has been administered. Encourage patient to retain solution at least 5 minutes. ☐ ☐ _____

18. When patient is no longer able to retain solution, assist patient to bedpan, bedside commode, or bathroom. ☐ ☐ _____

19. Instruct patient to call to inspect results before stool is flushed. Observe characteristics of feces or solution. When enemas are ordered "until clear" in preparation for surgery, enemas are repeated until patient passes fluid that is clear and contains no fecal matter. Usually three consecutive enemas are adequate. If after three enemas the water is highly colored or contains solid fecal material, notify the nurse before continuing. ☐ ☐ _____

20. Promote patient involvement as much as possible. ☐ ☐ _____

	S	U	Comments
21. Determine the patient's tolerance of the procedure, being alert for signs and symptoms of discomfort and fatigue. If the patient cannot tolerate a procedure, describe this inability in the nursing notes.	☐	☐	_____
22. Provide for patient hygiene; assist patient to bed or chair.	☐	☐	_____
23. Document the following:			
Date and time	☐	☐	_____
Type and volume of enema	☐	☐	_____
Temperature of solution	☐	☐	_____
Characteristics of results	☐	☐	_____
How patient tolerated procedure	☐	☐	_____
24. Assist the patient to a position of comfort, and place needed items within easy reach. Ensure that the patient has a means to call for help and knows how to use it.	☐	☐	_____
25. Raise the side rails, and lower the bed to the lowest position.	☐	☐	_____
26. Remove gloves and all protective barriers such as gown, goggles, and masks. Store appropriately or discard. Remove and dispose of soiled supplies and equipment according to agency policy and guidelines from the CDC and OSHA.	☐	☐	_____
27. Perform hand hygiene after removing gloves.	☐	☐	_____
28. Document the patient's response to the procedure, expected or unexpected outcomes, and all patient teaching.	☐	☐	_____
29. Report any unexpected outcomes.	☐	☐	_____

PROCEDURE 23-2

PERFORMING COLOSTOMY AND ILEOSTOMY CARE

	S	U	Comments

Ostomy Care

1. Check the health care provider's order. ☐ ☐ _____

2. Introduce yourself to the patient; include your name and title or role. ☐ ☐ _____

3. Identify the patient by checking his or her identification bracelet and requesting that the patient state his or her name or birth date, or both. ☐ ☐ _____

4. Explain the procedure and the reason it is to be done in terms that the patient is able to understand. Advise the patient of any unpleasantness that may be involved with the procedure. Give the patient time to ask questions. ☐ ☐ _____

5. Determine need for and provide patient education before and during procedure. ☐ ☐ _____

6. Evaluate the patient. ☐ ☐ _____

7. Perform hand hygiene and don clean gloves according to agency policy and guidelines from the Centers for Disease Control and Prevention(CDC) and the Occupational Safety and Health Administration (OSHA). ☐ ☐ _____

8. Assemble equipment and complete necessary charges. ☐ ☐ _____

9. Prepare the patient for the procedure:

   a. Close the door or pull the privacy curtain around the patient's bed. ☐ ☐ _____

   b. Raise the bed to a comfortable working height, and lower the side rail on the side nearest the patient care technician. ☐ ☐ _____

   c. Position and drape the patient as necessary. ☐ ☐ _____

10. Observe for the following:

    a. Pouch leakage and length of time in place (Pouches must be changed every 3 to 7 days to prevent skin impairment.) ☐ ☐ _____

    b. Stoma for healing and color (Proper stoma appearance is moist and reddish pink.) ☐ ☐ _____

	S	U	Comments

c. Abdominal incision   ☐ ☐ _____

11. Arrange supplies and equipment at patient's bedside or in bathroom.   ☐ ☐ _____

12. Position patient supine and comfortable.   ☐ ☐ _____

13. Carefully remove wafer seal from skin (adhesive solvent is sometimes needed).   ☐ ☐ _____

14. Place reusable pouch in bedpan or disposable pouch in plastic bag.   ☐ ☐ _____

15. Cleanse skin around stoma with warm water; pat dry.   ☐ ☐ _____

16. Measure stoma opening.   ☐ ☐ _____

17. Place toilet tissue over stoma; use gauze for ileostomy. Note color and viability of stoma. If skin sealant is to be used, apply to skin and allow to dry.   ☐ ☐ _____

18. Apply protective skin barrier about 1/16 inch from stoma.   ☐ ☐ _____

19. Cut an opening in the center of wafer to 1/16 inch larger than stoma, and apply protective wafer with flange.   ☐ ☐ _____

20. Gently attach pouch to flange by compressing the two together.   ☐ ☐ _____

21. Remove tissue or gauze from stoma and backing from protectant wafer; center opening over stoma, and press against skin for 1 to 2 minutes.   ☐ ☐ _____

22. Fold over bottom edges of pouch once to fit clamp. Secure clamp. If bottom edge of pouch is folded over more than once, the plastic will be too thick for the clamp, thus springing the clamp and causing spillage of fecal matter.   ☐ ☐ _____

23. If patient uses belt, attach at this time.   ☐ ☐ _____

24. Assist patient to comfortable position in bed or chair; remove equipment from bedside.   ☐ ☐ _____

25. Empty, wash, and dry reusable pouch.   ☐ ☐ _____

26. Promote patient involvement as much as possible.   ☐ ☐ _____

27. Determine the patient's tolerance of the procedure, being alert for signs and symptoms of discomfort and fatigue. If the patient cannot tolerate a procedure, describe this inability in the nursing notes.   ☐ ☐ _____

	S	U	Comments
28. Document the following:	☐	☐	_____
Date and time	☐	☐	_____
Procedure	☐	☐	_____
Type of pouch	☐	☐	_____
Type of skin barrier	☐	☐	_____
Amount and appearance of feces	☐	☐	_____
Condition of stoma and peristomal skin	☐	☐	_____
Patient's level of participation	☐	☐	_____
29. Assist the patient to a position of comfort, and place needed items within easy reach. Ensure that the patient has a means to call for help and knows how to use it.	☐	☐	_____
30. Raise the side rails, and lower the bed to the lowest position.	☐	☐	_____
31. Remove gloves and all protective barriers such as gown, goggles, and masks. Store appropriately or discard. Remove and dispose of soiled supplies and equipment according to agency policy and guidelines from the CDC and OSHA.	☐	☐	_____
32. Perform hand hygiene after removing gloves.	☐	☐	_____
33. Document the patient's response to the procedure,expected or unexpected outcomes, and all patient teaching.	☐	☐	_____
34. Report any unexpected outcomes.	☐	☐	_____

This page intentionally left blank

PROCEDURE 24-1

ASSISTING WITH DEEP-BREATHING AND COUGHING EXERCISES

	S	U	Comments
1. Verify with the nurse the procedure to be performed.	☐	☐	_____
2. Introduce yourself to the patient; include your name and title or role.	☐	☐	_____
3. Identify the patient by checking his or her identification bracelet and requesting that the patient state his or her name or birth date, or both.	☐	☐	_____
4. Explain the procedure and the reason it is to be done in terms that the patient is able to understand. Advise the patient of anything uncomfortable that may be involved with the procedure. Give the patient time to ask questions.	☐	☐	_____
5. Determine need for and provide patient education before and during procedure. Notify the nurse of any additional educational needs.	☐	☐	_____
6. Perform hand hygiene and don clean gloves according to agency policy and guidelines from the Centers for Disease Control and Prevention(CDC) and the Occupational Safety and Health Administration (OSHA).	☐	☐	_____
7. Assemble equipment, and complete necessary charges.	☐	☐	_____
8. Prepare the patient for the procedure:			
a. Close the door or pull the privacy curtain around the patient's bed.	☐	☐	_____
b. Raise the bed to a comfortable working height, and lower the side rail on the side nearest the patient care technician.	☐	☐	_____
c. Position and drape the patient as necessary. Descriptions of specific positions are included in each procedure.	☐	☐	_____
9. Assist patient to a semi-Fowler's position or sitting on the side of the bed or standing position. (Upright positions facilitate diaphragmatic movement.)	☐	☐	_____
10. Stand or sit facing the patient. (Allows patient to observe the breathing exercise.)	☐	☐	_____

	S	U	Comments

11. Instruct the patient to place palms of hands across from each other, down and along lower borders of the anterior rib cage. Place tips of fingers lightly together. ☐ ☐ _____

12. Show patient how to take slow, deep breaths, inhaling through nose and pushing abdomen against hands. Have him or her feel middle fingers separate during inhalation. Explain that the patient will feel normal downward movement of the diaphragm while inhaling and that abdominal organs move down and chest wall expands. ☐ ☐ _____

13. Instruct patient to avoid using chest and shoulders while inhaling. ☐ ☐ _____

14. Repeat complete breathing exercise 3 to 5 times. ☐ ☐ _____

15. Have patient practice exercise. Instruct him or her to take 10 slow, deep breaths every hour while awake. ☐ ☐ _____

16. Next, explain the importance of maintaining an upright or sitting position for the patient to be able to produce an effective cough. ☐ ☐ _____

17. If the patient has a surgical incision on either the throat or abdomen, teach the patient to place a pillow or bath blanket over the incisional area and place hands over pillow to splint the incision. During breathing and coughing exercises, have the patient press gently against the incisional area for splinting and support. ☐ ☐ _____

18. Demonstrate coughing. Instruct patient to take two slow, deep breaths, inhaling through nose and exhaling through mouth. ☐ ☐ _____

19. Show the patient how to inhale deeply a third time and hold breath to a count of three. Cough fully for two or three coughs without inhaling between coughs. Tell the patient to push all air out of the lungs. ☐ ☐ _____

20. Caution patient against just clearing his/her throat instead of coughing. ☐ ☐ _____

21. Have patient practice coughing exercises 2 to 3 times every 2 hours while awake. ☐ ☐ _____

22. Instruct patient to look at sputum, or mucus, each time for consistency, odor, amount, and color changes. Have the patient report any noted changes to either you or the nurse. ☐ ☐ _____

PROCEDURE 24-2

OXYGEN ADMINISTRATION

	S	U	Comments
1. Verify with the nurse the procedure to be done.	☐	☐	_____
2. Introduce yourself to the patient; include your name and title or role.	☐	☐	_____
3. Identify the patient by checking his or her identification bracelet and requesting that the patient state his or her name or birth date, or both.	☐	☐	_____
4. Explain the procedure and the reason it is to be done in terms that the patient is able to understand. Advise the patient of anything uncomfortable that may be involved with the procedure. Give the patient time to ask questions.	☐	☐	_____
5. Determine need for and provide patient education before and during procedure. Notify the nurse of any additional educational needs.	☐	☐	_____
6. Perform hand hygiene and don clean gloves according to agency policy and guidelines from the Centers for Disease Control and Prevention (CDC) and the Occupational Safety and Health Administration (OSHA).	☐	☐	_____
7. Assemble equipment, and complete necessary charges.	☐	☐	_____
8. Prepare the patient for the procedure:			
a. Close the door or pull the privacy curtain around the patient's bed.	☐	☐	_____
b. Raise the bed to a comfortable working height, and lower the side rail on the side nearest the patient care technician.	☐	☐	_____
c. Position and drape the patient as necessary. Descriptions of specific positions are included in each procedure.	☐	☐	_____
9. Assemble equipment.	☐	☐	_____
10. Explain necessary precautions during oxygen therapy.	☐	☐	_____
11. Position patient in Fowler's or semi-Fowler's position.	☐	☐	_____

	S	U	Comments

12. Auscultate lung sounds, and observe for signs and symptoms of hypoxia or respiratory distress. Review laboratory reports of arterial blood gas levels. Suction any secretions obstructing the airway, and listen to lung sounds after suctioning (see Procedure 24.4). ☐ ☐ _____

13. Fill humidifier container to designated level. Humidify oxygen if flow rate is greater than 4 L/min. Use only sterile water in humidifier. ☐ ☐ _____

14. Attach flowmeter to humidifier, and insert in proper oxygen source: central oxygen outlet, portable oxygen cylinder, or oxygen concentrator. Verify that water is bubbling. ☐ ☐ _____

15. Administer oxygen therapy:

   a. Nasal cannula: A simple, two-pronged plastic device that is used to deliver low concentrations of oxygen. A nasal cannula allows patient to eat and talk normally, and its use is appropriate for all age groups. ☐ ☐ _____

   (1) Attach nasal cannula tubing to flowmeter. ☐ ☐ _____

   (2) Adjust flowmeter to 6 to 10 L/min to flush tubing and prongs with oxygen. ☐ ☐ _____

   (3) Adjust flow rate to prescribed amount; 1 to 6 L/min may be ordered. ☐ ☐ _____

   (4) Place a nasal prong into each nostril of the patient. ☐ ☐ _____

   (5) Place cannula tubing over the patient's ears, and tighten under the chin. ☐ ☐ _____

   (6) Place padding between strap and ears if needed. Use lambswool, gauze, or cotton balls. ☐ ☐ _____

   (7) Ensure that the cannula tubing is long enough to allow for patient movement. ☐ ☐ _____

   (8) Regularly evaluate equipment and patient's respiratory status. ☐ ☐ _____

      (a) Evaluate cannula frequently for possible obstruction. ☐ ☐ _____

      (b) Observe external nasal area, nares, and superior surface of both ears for skin impairment every 6 to 8 hours. ☐ ☐ _____

	S	U	Comments

(c) Observe nares and cannula prongs at least once a shift for irritation or breakage. Cleanse skin with cotton-tipped applicator as needed. ☐ ☐ _____

(d) Apply water-soluble lubricant to nares if needed. ☐ ☐ _____

(e) Refer to the nurse for any prescribed changes in flow rate. ☐ ☐ _____

(f) Maintain solution in humidifier container, if used, at appropriate level at all times. ☐ ☐ _____

b. Face mask: Depending on patient's respiratory condition, the health care provider may prescribe delivery of oxygen mask. The mask is designed to fit snugly over the patient's nose and mouth. Different types of masks are used according to patient's needs, such as the Venturi mask, the partial-rebreathing mask, the non-rebreathing mask, and the simple face mask.

(1) Adjust flow rate of oxygen according to what the nurse told you. Usually 6 to 10 L/min, which is measured in percentages (35% to 95%), is prescribed. In some facilities, the respiratory therapist assumes responsibility for maintaining proper flow. Observe for fine mist or bubbling in humidifier. ☐ ☐ _____

(2) Explain to the patient the need for oxygen mask. ☐ ☐ _____

(3) Allow patient to hold the oxygen mask over the bridge of the nose and mouth, if he or she is able. Assist as necessary. ☐ ☐ _____

(4) Adjust straps around patient's head and over ears. Place cotton ball or gauze over ears under elastic straps. ☐ ☐ _____

(5) Observe reservoir bag for appropriate movement if one is attached to mask. ☐ ☐ _____

(a) Partial-rebreathing mask: When functioning properly, the reservoir fills on exhalation and almost collapses on inhalation.

(b) Non-rebreathing mask: When functioning properly, the reservoir, or bag fills on exhalation but never totally collapses on inhalation.

(6) Evaluate equipment function regularly.

	S	U	Comments

(a) Remove mask and evaluate skin every 2 to 4 hours. Clean and dry skin as needed. ☐ ☐ _____

(b) Refer to the nurse for prescribed flow rate and any changes. ☐ ☐ _____

(c) Maintain solution in humidifier container, if used, at appropriate level at all times. Always use sterile water, never tap water. ☐ ☐ _____

After the Procedure

16. Assist the patient to a position of comfort, and place needed items within easy reach. Ensure that the patient has a means to call for help and knows how to use it. ☐ ☐ _____

17. Raise the side rails, and lower the bed to the lowest position. ☐ ☐ _____

18. Remove gloves and all protective barriers such as gown, goggles, and masks. Store appropriately or discard. Remove and dispose of soiled supplies and equipment according to agency policy and guidelines from the CDC and OSHA. ☐ ☐ _____

19. Perform hand hygiene after removing gloves. ☐ ☐ _____

20. Report any unexpected outcomes to the nurse. Specific notes for reporting unexpected outcomes are included in each procedure. ☐ ☐ _____

21. Document the following:

Date ☐ ☐ _____

Time ☐ ☐ _____

Flow rate ☐ ☐ _____

Method of oxygen delivery ☐ ☐ _____

Evaluation of respiratory status ☐ ☐ _____

Patient's response to oxygen therapy ☐ ☐ _____

Changes in health care provider's orders ☐ ☐ _____

Adverse reactions or side effects of oxygen therapy ☐ ☐ _____

PROCEDURE 24-3

TRACHEOSTOMY SUCTIONING AND CARE

	S	U	Comments

1. Verify with the nurse the procedure to be done. ☐ ☐ _____

2. Introduce yourself to the patient; include your name and title or role. ☐ ☐ _____

3. Identify the patient by checking his or her identification bracelet and requesting that the patient state his or her name or birth date, or both. ☐ ☐ _____

4. Explain the procedure and the reason it is to be done in terms that the patient is able to understand. Advise the patient of anything uncomfortable that may be involved with the procedure. Give the patient time to ask questions. ☐ ☐ _____

5. Determine need for and provide patient education before and during procedure. Notify the nurse of any additional educational needs. ☐ ☐ _____

6. Perform hand hygiene and don clean gloves according to agency policy and guidelines from the Centers for Disease Control and Prevention (CDC) and the Occupational Safety and Health Administration (OSHA). ☐ ☐ _____

7. Assemble equipment, and complete necessary charges. ☐ ☐ _____

8. Prepare the patient for the procedure:

   a. Close the door or pull the privacy curtain around the patient's bed. ☐ ☐ _____

   b. Raise the bed to a comfortable working height, and lower the side rail on the side nearest the patient care technician ☐ ☐ _____

   c. Position and drape the patient as necessary. Descriptions of specific positions are included in each procedure. ☐ ☐ _____

9. Assemble equipment. ☐ ☐ _____

10. Check patient's tracheostomy for exudate, edema, and respiratory obstruction. ☐ ☐ _____

11. Position patient in semi-Fowler's position. ☐ ☐ _____

12. Provide paper and pencil or a communication board for patient. ☐ ☐ _____

267

	S	U	Comments

13. Position self at head of bed facing patient. Always face patient while cleaning or suctioning a tracheostomy. ☐ ☐ _____

14. Auscultate lung sounds. ☐ ☐ _____

15. Place towel or prepackaged drape under tracheostomy and across chest. ☐ ☐ _____

16. Perform hand hygiene. Prepare equipmentand supplies on over the bed table. Check suction equipment and machine. ☐ ☐ _____

    a. Open suction catheter kit but maintain sterility of contents, leaving the tip in its wrapper. Don sterile gloves. Open basin for sterile saline. Attach end of suction catheter to suction machine tubing, and pick up tubing from the machine with the nondominant hand. Fan fold or wrap suction catheter around dominant hand. ☐ ☐ _____

    b. Use nondominant hand to pour rinsing solution (sterile normal saline) into basin. ☐ ☐ _____

    c. Turn on suction machine with nondominant hand. ☐ ☐ _____

17. Preoxygenate patient by having patient take several deep breaths. If patient is receiving oxygen, wait to remove oxygen delivery system until just before suctioning. ☐ ☐ _____

18. Suction tracheal cannula.

    a. Place thumb over suction control vent; place tip of suction catheter in container of sterile rinse solution. Withdraw sterile rinsing solution through catheter by placing thumb over suction control. ☐ ☐ _____

    b. Remove thumb from suction control; advance catheter until resistance is met, and then withdraw catheter approximately 1 cm. (Depth of catheter approximately equals the length of outer cannula, the distal end of which protrudes from the opening approximately 1 to 2 inches.) ☐ ☐ _____

    c. Apply intermittent suction by placing thumb on and off suction control, and gently rotate catheter as it is withdrawn. ☐ ☐ _____

    d. Suction for a maximum of 10 seconds a ta time, never longer. ☐ ☐ _____

    e. Rinse catheter with sterile solution by suctioning sterile solution through it. Repeat steps 18b through 18d if needed. ☐ ☐ _____

	S	U	Comments

f. Allow patient to rest between each suctioning effort. If patient was previously receiving oxygen, reapply it at the prescribed rate between each suctioning episode. ☐ ☐ _____

g. Turn off suction, and dispose of catheter appropriately. Perform hand hygiene. ☐ ☐ _____

h. Auscultate lung sounds. ☐ ☐ _____

After the Procedure

19. Assist the patient to a position of comfort, and place needed items within easy reach. Ensure that the patient has a means to call for help and knows how to use it. ☐ ☐ _____

20. Raise the side rails, and lower the bed to the lowest position. ☐ ☐ _____

21. Remove gloves and all protective barriers such as gown, goggles, and masks. Store appropriately or discard. Remove and dispose of soiled supplies and equipment according to agency policy and guidelines from the CDC and OSHA. ☐ ☐ _____

22. Perform hand hygiene after removing gloves. ☐ ☐ _____

23. Report any unexpected outcomes to the nurse. Specific notes for reporting unexpected outcomes are included in each procedure. ☐ ☐ _____

24. Document the following:

Date ☐ ☐ _____

Time ☐ ☐ _____

Tracheostomy suctioned ☐ ☐ _____

Characteristics of material that was suctioned ☐ ☐ _____

Amount ☐ ☐ _____

Color ☐ ☐ _____

Consistency ☐ ☐ _____

Adverse reactions ☐ ☐ _____

Patient's response ☐ ☐ _____

If oxygen is administered, note flow rate and method used ☐ ☐ _____

	S	**U**	**Comments**

Tracheostomy Care

1. Refer to standard steps 1 to 9. ☐ ☐ _____

2. Check patient's tracheostomy for sanguineous exudate, edema, and respiratory obstruction. ☐ ☐ _____

3. Perform suctioning if it is needed before performing tracheostomy care. ☐ ☐ _____

4. Position patient in semi-Fowler's position. ☐ ☐ _____

5. Perform hand hygiene; then position self at head of bed, facing patient. Always face patient while cleaning or suctioning a tracheostomy. ☐ ☐ _____

6. Don, or put on, clean glove on nondominanthand. Remove old dressing from around tracheostomy stoma, and discard it in appropriate receptacle. ☐ ☐ _____

7. Prepare equipment and supplies. ☐ ☐ _____

   a. Open tracheostomy cleaning kit with aseptic technique. ☐ ☐ _____

   b. If basins are packed with sterile gloves, apply one sterile glove to dominant hand. Separate basins with dominant hand. Use nondominant hand to pour cleansing solution (hydrogen peroxide) in one basin and rinsing solution (sterile saline) in another basin. In some facilities, a third solution of half hydrogen peroxide and half normal saline is used to clean around the tracheostomy stoma. Check facility policy. ☐ ☐ _____

8. With nondominant hand, unlock and remove inner cannula; place in hydrogen peroxide cleansing solution. Never remove outer cannula. If it is expelled by patient, use hemostat to hold tracheostomy open and call for assistance. Always have a sterile packaged hemostat, as well as an extra sterile tracheostomy set, available at bedside. ☐ ☐ _____

9. Apply second sterile glove, or apply new pair of sterile gloves if contamination has occurred. ☐ ☐ _____

10. Clean inner cannula.

    a. Use brush to clean inside and outside of inner cannula. ☐ ☐ _____

    b. Place inner cannula in sterile normal saline solution. ☐ ☐ _____

    c. At some facilities, pipe cleaners are used to dry inside of inner cannula. Check facility policy. ☐ ☐ _____

	S	U	Comments
d. Inspect inner and outer areas of inner cannula. Remove excess liquid.	☐	☐	_____
e. Insert inner cannula and lock in place.	☐	☐	_____
11. Clean skin around tracheostomy and tabs of outer cannula with hydrogen peroxide (orhalf-and-half mixture) and cotton-tipped swabs; clean away from the opening. Use wipes tha tare free of lint around the tracheostomy opening.	☐	☐	_____
12. It may be necessary to rinse cleansing solution from skin. If so, use sterile 4 × 4 gauze. Place dry, sterile dressing around tracheostomy faceplate.	☐	☐	_____
13. Change cotton tapes holding tracheostomyin place if necessary.	☐	☐	_____
a. If assistance is not available, thread clean tie through opening in flange of outer cannula alongside old tie. If assistance is available, untie one side of cotton tape from outer cannula and replace with clean one while the assistant stabilizes thetracheostomy tube.	☐	☐	_____
b. Bring clean tape under back of neck.	☐	☐	_____
c. If assistance is not available, thread tie through opening in opposite flange of outer cannula alongside old tie. If assistance is available, remove other side from outer cannula and replace with clean tape.	☐	☐	_____
d. Tie ends of clean cotton tapes together in a knot at side of neck.	☐	☐	_____
14. Auscultate lung sounds.	☐	☐	_____
15. Provide mouth care.	☐	☐	_____

After the Procedure

	S	U	Comments
16. Assist the patient to a position of comfort,and place needed items within easy reach. Ensure that the patient has a means to call for help and knows how to use it.	☐	☐	_____
17. Raise the side rails, and lower the bed to the lowest position.	☐	☐	_____
18. Remove gloves and all protective barriers such as gown, goggles, and masks. Store appropriately or discard. Remove and dispose of soiled supplies and equipment according to agency policy and guidelines from the CDC and OSHA.	☐	☐	_____

	S	U	Comments
19. Perform hand hygiene after removing gloves.	☐	☐	_____
20. Report any unexpected outcomes to the nurse. Specific notes for reporting unexpected outcomes are included in each procedure.	☐	☐	_____
21. Place call light, paper, and pencil with ineasy reach of the patient.	☐	☐	_____
22. Reassess patient's tracheostomy for signs of bleeding, edema, and respiratory obstruction.	☐	☐	_____
23. Document the following:			
Date/time of tracheostomy care	☐	☐	_____
Type of tracheostomy care performed	☐	☐	_____
Patient's response	☐	☐	_____
Evaluation of respiratory status	☐	☐	_____
Adverse reactions	☐	☐	_____
Condition of tracheal stoma and peristomal skin	☐	☐	_____
If oxygen is administered, note flow rate and method used	☐	☐	_____

PROCEDURE 24-4

OROPHARYNGEAL SUCTIONING

	S	U	Comments
1. Verify with the nurse the procedure to be done.	☐	☐	_____
2. Introduce yourself to the patient; include your name and title or role.	☐	☐	_____
3. Identify the patient by checking his or her identification bracelet and requesting that the patient state his or her name or birth date, or both.	☐	☐	_____
4. Explain the procedure and the reason it is to be done in terms that the patient is able to understand. Advise the patient of anything uncomfortable that may be involved with the procedure. Give the patient time to ask questions.	☐	☐	_____
5. Determine need for and provide patient education before and during procedure. Notify the nurse of any additional educational needs.	☐	☐	_____
6. Perform hand hygiene and don clean gloves according to agency policy and guidelines from the Centers for Disease Control and Prevention (CDC) and the Occupational Safety and Health Administration (OSHA).	☐	☐	_____
7. Assemble equipment, and complete necessary charges.	☐	☐	_____
8. Prepare the patient for the procedure			
a. Close the door or pull the privacy curtain around the patient's bed.	☐	☐	_____
b. Raise the bed to a comfortable working height, and lower the side rail on the side nearest the patient care technician.	☐	☐	_____
c. Position and drape the patient as necessary. Descriptions of specific positions are included in each procedure.	☐	☐	_____
9. Assemble equipment.	☐	☐	_____
10. Evaluate need for suctioning.	☐	☐	_____
• Gurgling respirations	☐	☐	_____
• Restlessness	☐	☐	_____

	S	U	Comments
• Vomitus in mouth	☐	☐	_____
• Drooling	☐	☐	_____
11. Explain procedure to the patient and that coughing, sneezing, or gagging is expected.	☐	☐	_____
12. Position patient.	☐	☐	_____
a. If patient is alert and conscious, place in semi-Fowler's position with head to one side.	☐	☐	_____
b. If patient is unconscious, place in side-lying position facing you.	☐	☐	_____
(1) Place towel lengthwise under patient's chin and over pillow.	☐	☐	_____
13. Pour sterile normal saline solution into sterile container.	☐	☐	_____
14. Perform hand hygiene and don cleang loves. Turn on suction machine, and select appropriate suction pressure. (Check facility policy.) Never suction with any more vacuum pressure than needed to remove the secretions, and use the smallest catheter that will remove the secretions well. Connect suction catheter to tubing.	☐	☐	_____
a. Common vacuum settings for wall suction units:	☐	☐	_____
(1) Infants: 60 to 80 mm Hg	☐	☐	_____
(2) Children: 100 to 120 mm Hg	☐	☐	_____
(3) Adults: 120 to 150 mm Hg	☐	☐	_____
b. Common catheter sizes:	☐	☐	_____
(1) Infants: 6- to 8-Fr	☐	☐	_____
(2) Children: 10- to 12-Fr	☐	☐	_____
(3) Adults: 12- to 14-Fr	☐	☐	_____
15. Suction solution through catheter by placing thumb over open end of connector or over vent.	☐	☐	_____
16. Remove thumb from open end of connector or vent, or pinch catheter with thumb and index finger.	☐	☐	_____
17. Proceed with suctioning.	☐	☐	_____
a. Oropharyngeal suctioning:	☐	☐	_____
(1) Don clean gloves if those are not already on.	☐	☐	_____

	S	U	Comments

(2) Gently insert Yankauer or tonsillar tip suction catheter into one side of mouth and glide it toward oropharynx with outsuction. ☐ ☐ _____

(3) Place thumb over open end of connector or vet to apply suction. Move Yankauer or tonsillar tip catheter around mouth until secretions are cleared. ☐ ☐ _____

(4) Encourage patient to cough. ☐ ☐ _____

(5) Rinse Yankauer or tonsillar tip catheter with water in cup or basin until connecting tubing is cleared of secretions. Turn off suction. ☐ ☐ _____

(6) Repeat procedure as necessary. ☐ ☐ _____

18. Observe patient closely, and limit suction to 10 to 15 seconds. ☐ ☐ _____

19. Repeat suctioning if it is needed. ☐ ☐ _____

20. Allow 1 to 2 minutes of rest between suctioning if it is necessary to repeat procedure. If oxygen is administered by nasal cannula, mask, or other means, reapply oxygen during rest period. ☐ ☐ _____

21. If patient is alert and is able to cooperate, instruct patient to breathe deeply and cough between suctioning attempts. ☐ ☐ _____

22. When suctioning of catheter is complete, suction between cheeks and gum line and under tongue; suction mouth last to prevent contaminating catheter. ☐ ☐ _____

23. Place catheter in solution and apply suction. ☐ ☐ _____

24. Discard catheter and used suction catheters: wrap catheter around gloved hand; pull glove off hand and over catheter. Remove face shield, if worn. Perform hand hygiene. ☐ ☐ _____

25. Place sterile, unopened catheter at patient's bedside. ☐ ☐ _____

26. Provide mouth care. ☐ ☐ _____

27. Evaluate patient's breathing patterns, fatigue, vital signs, level of consciousness, and color. ☐ ☐ _____

28. Determine whether patient has a decrease in anxiety. ☐ ☐ _____

After the Procedure

29. Assist the patient to a position of comfort, and place needed items within easy reach. ☐ ☐ _____

275

	S	U	Comments
30. Ensure that the patient has a means to call for help and knows how to use it.	☐	☐	_____
31. Raise the side rails, and lower the bed to the lowest position.	☐	☐	_____
32. Remove gloves and all protective barriers such as gown, goggles, and masks. Store appropriately or discard. Remove and dispose of soiled supplies and equipment according to agency policy and guidelines from the CDC and OSHA.	☐	☐	_____
33. Perform hand hygiene after removing gloves.	☐	☐	_____
34. Report any unexpected outcomes to the nurse. Specific notes for reporting unexpected outcomes are included in each procedure.	☐	☐	_____
35. Place call light, paper, and pencil within easy reach of the patient.	☐	☐	_____
36. Document the following:			
Date	☐	☐	_____
Time	☐	☐	_____
Method of suctioning	☐	☐	_____
Amount, consistency, color, and odor of secretions	☐	☐	_____
Respiratory assessment before and after procedure	☐	☐	_____
Patient's response	☐	☐	_____

PROCEDURE 25-1

COLLECTING A VENOUS BLOOD SAMPLE WITH A SYRINGE

	S	U	Comments
1. Check the requisition form to determine the tests ordered. Gather the appropriate tube sand supplies.	☐	☐	_____
2. Perform hand hygiene and put on nonsterile gloves.	☐	☐	_____
3. Identify the patient, explain the procedure, and obtain permission to perform the venipuncture.	☐	☐	_____
4. Assist the patient to sit with the arm well supported in a slightly downward position.	☐	☐	_____
5. Assemble the equipment. The choice of syringe barrel size and needle size depends on your inspection of the patient's veins and the amount of blood required for the ordered tests. Attach the needle to the syringe. Pull and depress the plunger several times to loosen it in the barrel. Keep the cover on the needle.	☐	☐	_____
6. Apply the tourniquet around the patient's arm 3 to 4 inches above the puncture site. The tourniquet should never be tied so tightly that it restricts blood flow in the artery. The tourniquet should remain in place no longer than 120 seconds for the entire procedure.	☐	☐	_____
7. Ask the patient to make a fist.	☐	☐	_____
8. Select the venipuncture site by palpating the antecubital space (if you have difficulty palpating the vein with gloves, you can remove the gloves, palpate the vein andvisibly mark its location, then put on new gloves before continuing); use your index finger to trace the path of the vein and to judge its depth. The vein most often used is the median cephalic vein, which lies in the middle of the elbow.	☐	☐	_____
9. Cleanse the site, starting in the center of the area and working outward in a circular pattern spiraling outward with friction, using an alcohol pad of 70% isopropyl alcohol or other antiseptic. Tourniquet may be released during this time.	☐	☐	_____
10. Allow the area to dry before proceeding. Reapply the tourniquet.	☐	☐	_____

	S	U	Comments

11. Hold the syringe in your dominant hand. Your thumb should be on top and your fingers underneath. Remove the needle sheath. ☐ ☐ _____

12. Grasp the patient's arm with the nondominanth and and anchor the vein by stretching the skin downward below the collection site with the thumb of the nondominant hand. ☐ ☐ _____

13. With the bevel of the needle up, aligned parallel to the vein, and at a 15-degree angle, insert the needle through the skin and into the in one quick and smooth motion. Observe for a "flash" of blood in the hub of the syringe. Ask the patient to release the fist. ☐ ☐ _____

14. Slowly pull back the plunger of the syringe with the nondominant hand. Do not allow more than 1 mL of head space between the blood and the top of the plunger. Make sure you do not move the needle after entering the vein. Fill the barrel to the needed volume. ☐ ☐ _____

15. Release the tourniquet when venipuncture is complete. It must be released before the needle is removed from the arm. ☐ ☐ _____

16. Place sterile gauze over the puncture site at the time of needle withdrawal. Immediately activate the needle safety device. ☐ ☐ _____

17. Instruct the patient to apply direct pressure on the puncture site with sterile gauze. The patient may elevate the arm but should not bend it. ☐ ☐ _____

18. Transfer the blood immediately to the required tube or tubes using a safety syringe transfer adapter. Do not push on the plunger during transfer. Discard the entire unit in the sharps container when transfer is complete. Invert the tubes after the addition of blood and label them with the necessary patient information. ☐ ☐ _____

19. Inspect the puncture site for bleeding or hematoma. ☐ ☐ _____

20. Apply a hypoallergenic bandage. ☐ ☐ _____

21. Disinfect the work area, dispose of any blood-contaminated materials (e.g., gauze) in the biohazard container, remove yourg loves, and sanitize your hands. ☐ ☐ _____

22. Complete the laboratory requisition form and route the specimen to the proper place. Record the procedure in the patient's record. ☐ ☐ _____

PROCEDURE 25-2

COLLECTING A VENOUS BLOOD SAMPLE USING AN EVACUATED TUBE

	S	U	Comments
1. Check the requisition form to determine the tests ordered. Gather the appropriate tube sand supplies.	☐	☐	_____
2. Perform hand hygiene and put on nonsterile gloves.	☐	☐	_____
3. Identify the patient, explain the procedure, and obtain permission for the venipuncture.	☐	☐	_____
4. Assist the patient to sit with the arm well supported in a slightly downward position.	☐	☐	_____
5. Assemble the equipment. The choice of needle size depends on your inspection of the patient's veins. Attach the needle firmly to the Vacutainer holder. Keep the cover on the needle.	☐	☐	_____
6. Apply the tourniquet around the patient's arm 3 to 4 inches above the puncture site. The tourniquet should never be tied so tightly that it restricts blood flow in the artery. Tourniquets should remain in place no longer than 120 seconds during vein selection.	☐	☐	_____
7. Ask the patient to make a fist.	☐	☐	_____
8. Select the venipuncture site by palpating the antecubital space and use your index finger to trace the path of the vein and to judge its depth. The vein most often used is the median cephalic vein, which lies in the middle of the elbow.	☐	☐	_____
9. Cleanse the site, starting in the center of the area and working outward in a circular spiraling outward with friction, using an alcohol pad of 70% isopropyl alcohol or other antiseptic. Tourniquet may be released during this time.	☐	☐	_____
10. Allow the site to dry for 0 to 60 seconds before proceeding.	☐	☐	_____
11. Reapply the tourniquet. Hold the Vacutainer assembly in your dominant hand. Your thumb should be on top and your fingers underneath. You may want to position the first tube to be drawn into the needle holder, but do not push it onto the double-pointed needle past the marking on the holder. Remove the needle sheath.	☐	☐	_____

	S	U	Comments

12. Grasp the patient's arm with the nondominanth and and anchor the vein by stretching the skin downward below the collection site with the thumb of the nondominant hand. ☐ ☐ _____

13. With the bevel of the needle up, aligned parallel to the vein, and at a 15-30-degree angle, insert the needle through the skin and into the vein in one quick and smooth motion. ☐ ☐ _____

14. Place two fingers on the flanges of the needle holder and use the thumb to push the tube onto the double-pointed needle. Make sure you do not change the needle's position in the vein. When blood begins to flow into the tube, ask the patient to release the fist. ☐ ☐ _____

15. Allow the tube to fill to maximum capacity. Remove the tube by curling the fingers underneath and pushing on the needle holder with the thumb. Take care not to move the needle when removing the tube. ☐ ☐ _____

16. Insert the second tube into the needle holder, following the instructions in the previous steps. Continue filling tubes until the order on the requisition has been filled. Gently invert each tube immediately after removing it from the needle holder to mix anticoagulants and blood. As the last tube is filling, release the tourniquet. ☐ ☐ _____

17. Remove the last tube from the holder. Place gauze over the puncture site and quickly remove the needle, engaging the safety device. Dispose of the entire unit in the sharps container. ☐ ☐ _____

18. Apply pressure to the gauze or instruct the patient to do so. The patient may elevate the arm but should not bend it. ☐ ☐ _____

19. Label the tubes with the patient's name, the date, and the time, or apply the preprinted tube labels. ☐ ☐ _____

20. Check the puncture site for bleeding and hematoma formation. ☐ ☐ _____

21. Apply a hypoallergenic bandage. ☐ ☐ _____

22. Disinfect the work area, dispose of any blood-contaminated materials (e.g., gauze) in the biohazard container, remove your gloves, and sanitize your hands. ☐ ☐ _____

23. Complete the laboratory requisition form and route the specimen to the proper place. Record the procedure in the patient's record. ☐ ☐ _____

PROCEDURE 25-3

COLLECTING CAPILLARY BLOOD USING DERMAL PUNCTURE

	S	U	Comments
1. Read the requisition and gather all needed supplies on the basis of the provider's requisition.	☐	☐	_____
2. Perform hand hygiene. Put on nonsterile gloves.	☐	☐	_____
3. Identify the patient and explain the procedure.	☐	☐	_____
4. Select a puncture site depending on the patient's age and the sample to be obtained (side of middle or ring finger of nondominant hand, medial or lateral curved surface of the heel for an infant).	☐	☐	_____
5. Gently rub the finger along the sides.	☐	☐	_____
6. Clean the site with alcohol, allow it to air dry, or dry it with sterile gauze.	☐	☐	_____
7. Grasp the patient's finger on the sides near the puncture site with your nondominant forefinger and thumb. Hold the lancet perpendicular to the patient's finger and make a rapid, deep puncture on the side of the patient's fingertip.	☐	☐	_____
8. Dispose of the lancet in the sharps container.	☐	☐	_____
9. Wipe away the first drop of blood with clean, sterile gauze.	☐	☐	_____
10. Apply gentle pressure to cause the blood to flow freely.	☐	☐	_____
11. Collect blood samples.			
a. Express a large drop of blood, touch the end of the tube to the drop of blood (not the finger), fill the capillary tubes, place the finger over the blood-free end of the tube, and seal the other end of the tube by inserting it into the sealing clay. The tube should be approximately three-quarters full before it is sealed.	☐	☐	_____
b. Wipe the finger with a clean, sterile gauze pad, express another large drop of blood, and fill a Microtainer®. Do not touch the container to the finger. If more blood is needed, wipe the puncture with clean gauze and gently squeeze another drop. Cap the tube when the collection is complete.	☐	☐	_____

	S	U	Comments

12. When collection is complete, apply pressure to the site with clean sterile gauze. The patient may be able to assist with this step. ☐ ☐ _____

13. Select an appropriate means of labeling the containers. ☐ ☐ _____

14. Capillary tubes can be placed in a red-topped tube, which is subsequently labeled. Microtainers® can be placed in zipper-lock bags that are subsequently labeled. ☐ ☐ _____

15. Check the patient for bleeding, clean the site if traces of blood are visible, and apply a nonallergenic bandage if indicated. ☐ ☐ _____

16. Dispose of used materials in the proper containers. ☐ ☐ _____

17. Disinfect the work area. Dispose of any blood-contaminated materials (e.g., gauze) in the biohazard container. Remove your gloves and sanitize your hands. ☐ ☐ _____

18. Record the procedure in the patient's record. ☐ ☐ _____

PROCEDURE 25-4

MEASURING BLOOD GLUCOSE

	S	U	Comments

1. Check the provider's order and collect the necessary equipment and supplies. Perform quality control measures according to the manufacturer's guidelines and facility policy. ☐ ☐ _____

2. Perform hand hygiene and put on gloves. ☐ ☐ _____

3. Ask the patient to wash his or her hands in warm soapy water and then rinse them in warm water and dry them completely. ☐ ☐ _____

4. Check the patient's index and ring fingers and select the site for puncture. ☐ ☐ _____

5. Turn on the Accu-Chek® monitor by pressing the ON button. ☐ ☐ _____

6. Make sure the code number on the LED display matches the code number on the container of test strips. ☐ ☐ _____

7. Remove a test strip from the vial and immediately replace the vial cover. ☐ ☐ _____

8. Check the strip for discoloration by comparing the color of the round window on the back of the test strip with the designated "unused" color chart provided on the label of the test strip vial. ☐ ☐ _____

9. Do not touch the yellow test pad or round window on the back of the strip when handling the strip. ☐ ☐ _____

10. When the test strip symbol begins flashing in the lower right corner of the display screen, insert the test strip into the designated testing slot until it locks into place. If the test strip has been inserted correctly, the arrows on the test strip will face up and point toward the monitor. ☐ ☐ _____

11. Cleanse the selected site on the patient's fingertip with the alcohol wipe and allow the finger to air-dry. ☐ ☐ _____

12. Perform the finger puncture and wipe away the first drop of blood. ☐ ☐ _____

13. Apply a large, hanging drop of blood to the center of the yellow testing pad. ☐ ☐ _____

    Do not touch the pad with the patient's finger. ☐ ☐ _____

	S	U	Comments
Do not apply a second drop of blood.	☐	☐	_____
Do not smear the blood with your finger.	☐	☐	_____
Make sure the yellow test pad is saturated with blood.	☐	☐	_____
14. Give the patient a gauze square to hold securely over the puncture site.	☐	☐	_____
15. The monitor automatically begins the measurement process as soon as it senses the drop of blood.	☐	☐	_____
16. The test result will be shown in the display window in milligrams per deciliter (mg/dL).	☐	☐	_____
17. Turn off the monitor by pressing the O button.	☐	☐	_____
18. Discard all biohazardous waste in the proper waste containers.	☐	☐	_____
19. Clean the glucometer according to the manufacturer's guidelines, disinfect the work area, remove your gloves and dispose of them properly, and sanitize your hands.	☐	☐	_____
20. Record the test results in the patient's electronic medical record.	☐	☐	_____

PROCEDURE 26-1

COLLECTION OF A 24-HOUR URINE SPECIMEN

	S	U	Comments
1. Greet the patient by name.	☐	☐	_____
2. Label the container with the patient's name and the current date, identify the specimen as a 24-hour urine specimen, and include your initials.	☐	☐	_____
3. Explain the following instructions to adult patients or to the guardians of pediatric patients.	☐	☐	_____
4. After explaining the following instructions, give the patient the specimen container with written instructions to confirm understanding.	☐	☐	_____

Patient Instructions for Obtaining a 24-Hour Urine Specimen

	S	U	Comments
5. Empty your bladder into the toilet in the morning without saving any of the specimen. Record the time you first emptied your bladder.	☐	☐	_____
6. For the next 24 hours, each time you empty your bladder, the urine should be voided directly into the large specimen container.	☐	☐	_____
7. Put the lid back on the container after each urination and store the container in the refrigerator or in an ice chest throughout the 24 hours of the study.	☐	☐	_____
8. If at any time you forget to empty your bladder into the specimen container, or if some urine is accidentally spilled, the test must be started all over again with an empty container and a newly recorded start time.	☐	☐	_____
9. The last collection of urine should be done at the same time as the first specimen on the previous day so that exactly 24 hours of urine collection is completed. The collection ends with the first voided morning specimen that completes the 24-hour collection period.	☐	☐	_____
10. As soon as possible after collection is completed, notify the nurse.	☐	☐	_____
11. Document the details of the patient education intervention in the patient's record.	☐	☐	_____

	S	U	Comments

Processing a 24-Hour Urine Specimen

1. Ask the patient whether he or she collected all voided urine throughout the 24-hour period or whether any problems occurred during the collection process.   ☐ ☐ _____

2. Complete the laboratory request form and prepare the specimen for transport.   ☐ ☐ _____

3. Store the specimen in the refrigerator until it is picked up by the laboratory.   ☐ ☐ _____

4. Document that the specimen was sent to the laboratory, including the type of test ordered, the date and time, and the type of specimen.   ☐ ☐ _____

PROCEDURE 26-2

COLLECTING A CLEAN-CATCH MIDSTREAM URINE SPECIMEN

	S	U	Comments
1. Label the container and give the patient the supplies.	☐	☐	_____
2. Explain the following instructions to adult patients or to the guardians of pediatric patients, being sensitive to privacy issues.	☐	☐	_____

Obtaining a Clean-Catch Midstream Specimen (Female Patients)

	S	U	Comments
3. Wash your hands and open the towelette packages for easy access.	☐	☐	_____
4. Remove the lid from the specimen container, being careful not to touch the inside of the lid or the inside of the container. Place the lid, facing up, on a paper towel.	☐	☐	_____
5. Remove your underclothing and sit on the toilet.	☐	☐	_____
6. Expose the urinary meatus by spreading a part the labia with one hand.	☐	☐	_____
7. Cleanse each side of the urinary meatus with a front-to-back motion, from the pubis to the anus. Use a separate antiseptic wipe to cleanse each side of the meatus.	☐	☐	_____
8. Cleanse directly across the meatus, front-to-back, using a third antiseptic wipe.	☐	☐	_____
9. Hold the labia apart throughout this procedure.	☐	☐	_____
10. Void a small amount of urine into the toilet.	☐	☐	_____
11. Move the specimen container into position and void the next portion of urine into it. Fill the container halfway. Remember, this is a sterile container. Do not put your fingers on the inside of the container.	☐	☐	_____
12. Remove the cup and void the last amount of urine into the toilet. (This means that the first part and the last part of the urinary flow have been excluded from the specimen. Only the middle portion of the flow is included.)	☐	☐	_____

	S	U	Comments

13. Place the lid on the container, taking care not to touch the interior surface of the lid. Wipe in your usual manner, redress, and return the sterile specimen to the place designated by the medical facility.   □   □ _____

Obtaining a Clean-Catch Midstream Specimen (Male Patients)

14. Wash your hands and expose the penis.   □   □ _____

15. Retract the foreskin of the penis (if not circumcised).   □   □ _____

16. Cleanse the area around the glans penis (meatus) and the urethral opening by washing each side of the glans with a separate antiseptic wipe.   □   □ _____

17. Cleanse directly across the urethral opening using a third antiseptic wipe.   □   □ _____

18. Void a small amount of urine into the toilet or urinal.   □   □ _____

19. Collect the next portion of the urine in the sterile container, filling the container halfway without touching the inside of the container with the hands or the penis.   □   □ _____

20. Void the last amount of urine into the toilet or urinal.   □   □ _____

21. Place the lid on the container, taking care not to touch the interior surface of the lid. Wipe and redress.   □   □ _____

22. Return the specimen to the designated area.   □   □ _____

Processing a Clean-Catch Urine Specimen

23. Document the date, time, and collection type.   □   □ _____

24. Process the specimen according to the provider's orders. Perform urinalysis in the office or prepare the specimen for transport to the laboratory. If it is to be sent to an outside laboratory, complete the following steps:

    a. Make sure the label is properly completed with patient information, date, time, and test ordered.   □   □ _____

    b. Place the specimen in a biohazard specimen bag.   □   □ _____

    c. Complete a laboratory requisition and place it in the outside pocket of the specimen bag.   □   □ _____

    d. Keep the specimen refrigerated until pickup.   □   □ _____

    e. Document that the specimen was sent.   □   □ _____

Student Name_____ Date_____

PROCEDURE 26-3

COLLECTING A URINE SPECIMEN FROM AN INFANT OR CHILD

	S	U	Comments
1. Assemble all needed supplies.	☐	☐	_____
2. Sanitize your hands and put on gloves.	☐	☐	_____
3. Ask the parent to remove the child's diaper or place the child in a supine position on the examination table and remove the diaper.	☐	☐	_____
4. Cleanse the genitalia with antiseptic wipes. Male: Cleanse the urinary meatus in a circular motion, starting directly on the meatus and working in an outward pattern. Repeat with a clean wipe. If the child has not been circumcised, gently retract the foreskin to expose the meatus; when you have completed the cleansing, return the foreskin to its natural position. Female: Hold the labia open with your nondominant hand; with your dominant hand, cleanse the inner labia, from the clitoris to the vaginal meatus, in a superior to inferior pattern. Discard the first wipe and repeat with a clean wipe, cleaning both sides of the inner labia.	☐	☐	_____
5. Make sure the area is dry. Unfold the collection device, remove the paper from the upper portion, place this portion over the mons pubis, and press it securely into place. Continue by removing the lower portion of the paper and securing this portion against the perineum. Make sure the device is attached smoothly and that you have not taped it to part of the infant's thigh.	☐	☐	_____
6. Rediaper the infant or, if the parent is helping, have the parent rediaper the infant at this time. The diaper will help hold the bag in place.	☐	☐	_____
7. Suggest that the parent give the child liquids, if allowed; check the bag for urine at frequent intervals.	☐	☐	_____
8. When a noticeable amount of urine has collected in the bag, put on gloves, remove the device, cleanse the skin area where the device was attached, and rediaper the child.	☐	☐	_____
9. Pour the urine carefully into the laboratory urine container and handle the sample in a routine manner.	☐	☐	_____

	S	U	Comments

10. Dispose of all used equipment in a biohazard waste container. ☐ ☐ _____

11. Remove your gloves, dispose of them in a biohazard container, and sanitize your hands. ☐ ☐ _____

12. Record the procedure in the patient's record. ☐ ☐ _____

PROCEDURE 26-4

TESTING URINE WITH CHEMICAL REAGENT STRIPS

	S	U	Comments
1. Sanitize your hands. Put on nonsterile gloves and eye protection.	☐	☐	_____
2. Check the time of collection, the container, and the mode of preservation.	☐	☐	_____
3. If the specimen has been refrigerated, allow it to warm to room temperature.	☐	☐	_____
4. Check the reagent strip container for the expiration date.	☐	☐	_____
5. Remove the reagent strip from the container. Hold it in your hand or place it on a clean paper towel. Recap the container tightly.	☐	☐	_____
6. Compare nonreactive test pads with the negative color blocks on the color chart on the container.	☐	☐	_____
7. Thoroughly mix the specimen by swirling.	☐	☐	_____
8. Following the manufacturer's directions, note the time, dip the strip into the urine, and then remove it.	☐	☐	_____
9. Quickly remove the excess urine from the strip by touching the side of the strip to a paper towel or to the side of the urine container.	☐	☐	_____
10. Hold the strip horizontally. At the required time, compare the strip with the appropriate color chart on the reagent container. Document on the reagent strip flow sheet each result as it is read. Alternately, the strip can be placed on a paper towel.	☐	☐	_____
11. Read the concentration by comparing the strip with the color chart on the side of the bottle.	☐	☐	_____
12. Clean the work area, remove your gloves, and sanitize your hands. If a paper towel was used, dispose of it, the reagent strip, and your gloves in the biohazard container.	☐	☐	_____
13. Document the results in the patient's record.	☐	☐	_____

This page intentionally left blank

PROCEDURE 26-5

COLLECTING A STOOL SPECIMEN

	S	U	Comments
1. Refer to the health care provider's order.	☐	☐	_____
2. Assemble supplies.	☐	☐	_____
3. Introduce self.	☐	☐	_____
4. Identify patient.	☐	☐	_____
5. Explain procedure to patient; make certain patient understands what is expected.	☐	☐	_____
6. Perform hand hygiene and don nonsterile gloves according to agency policy and guidelines from the CDC and OSHA.	☐	☐	_____
7. Assist patient to bathroom when necessary.	☐	☐	_____
8. Ask patient to defecate into commode, specimen device, or bedpan, preventing urine from entering specimen.	☐	☐	_____
9. Transfer stool to specimen cup with use of a tongue blade, and close the lid securely.	☐	☐	_____
10. Remove gloves, discard them in proper receptacle, and perform hand hygiene.	☐	☐	_____
11. Attach requisition slip, enclose in a biohazard bag, label the bag, and send specimen to laboratory (it is necessary to take specimens for ova and parasites to the laboratory stat; it is acceptable to keep other stool specimens at room temperature).	☐	☐	_____
12. Assist patient to bed.	☐	☐	_____
13. Document procedure and observations.	☐	☐	_____

This page intentionally left blank

PROCEDURE 26-6

COLLECTING A SPUTUM SPECIMEN BY EXPECTORATION

	S	U	Comments
1. Refer to the health care provider's order.	☐	☐	_____
2. Assemble supplies.			
3. Introduce self.	☐	☐	_____
4. Identify patient.	☐	☐	_____
5. Explain procedure.	☐	☐	_____
6. Perform hand hygiene and don nonsterile gloves according to agency policy and guidelines from the CDC and OSHA.	☐	☐	_____
7. Position patient in Fowler's position.	☐	☐	_____
8. Instruct patient to take three breaths and force cough into sterile container.	☐	☐	_____
9. Label specimen container.	☐	☐	_____
10. Enclose specimen in biohazard bag and attach laboratory requisition. Immediately send specimen to laboratory. If any sputum is present on outside of container, wash it off with disinfectant.	☐	☐	_____
11. Remove gloves, discard them in proper receptacle, and perform hand hygiene.	☐	☐	_____
12. Document procedure and observations.	☐	☐	_____

This page intentionally left blank

PROCEDURE 27-1

THE SURGICAL SKIN PREP

	S	U	Comments
1. Sanitize your hands.	☐	☐	_____
2. Instruct the patient in the skin preparation procedure, making sure the person understands the procedure and the rationale for it.	☐	☐	_____
3. Ask the patient to remove any clothing that might interfere with exposure of the site and provide a gown if needed.	☐	☐	_____
4. Assist the patient into the proper position for site exposure. Provide a drape if necessary to protect the patient's privacy.	☐	☐	_____
5. Expose the site. Use a light if necessary.	☐	☐	_____
6. Put on gloves and open the skin prep pack.	☐	☐	_____
7. Add the antiseptic soap to the two bowls.	☐	☐	_____
8. Start at the incision site and begin washing with the antiseptic soap on a gauze sponge in a circular motion, moving from the center to the edges of the area to be scrubbed.	☐	☐	_____
9. After one complete wipe, discard the sponge and begin again with a new sponge soaked in the antiseptic solution.	☐	☐	_____
10. When you return to the incision site for the next circular sweep, you must use clean material.	☐	☐	_____
11. Repeat the process, using sufficient friction for 5 minutes (or follow facility policy for the length of time required for a particular prep).	☐	☐	_____
12. If hair is present, the area may need to be clipped. Hold the skin taut and shave in the direction of growth. Take care to prevent injury to yourself or your patient. Immediately after completion, dispose of the razor in the sharps container.	☐	☐	_____
13. After shaving, scrub the skin a second time.	☐	☐	_____
14. Rinse the area with a sterile normal saline solution.	☐	☐	_____
15. Dry the area, using the same circular technique with dry sponges. The area may be dried by blotting with a sterile towel.	☐	☐	_____

	S	**U**	**Comments**
16. Paint on the antiseptic with the cotton-tipped applicators or gauze sponges, using the same circular technique and never returning to an area that has already been painted.	☐	☐	_____
17. Place a sterile drape and/or towel over the area.	☐	☐	_____
18. Answer all the patient's questions to relieve anxiety about the upcoming surgical procedure.	☐	☐	_____
19. Document completion of the skin prep in the patient's chart.	☐	☐	_____

PROCEDURE 27-2

APPLYING SEQUENTIAL COMPRESSION DEVICES

	S	U	Comments
1. Receive the request from the nurse to apply sequential compression stockings.	☐	☐	_____
2. Perform hand hygiene.	☐	☐	_____
3. The nurse may ask you to obtain baseline data about status of circulation such as the lower extremity pulses.	☐	☐	
4. Identify patient using two identifiers (i.e., name and birth date or name and account number, according to agency policy). Ask patient to state name.	☐	☐	
5. Perform hand hygiene. Provide hygiene to patient's lower extremities as needed.	☐	☐	_____
6. Assemble and prepare equipment.	☐	☐	_____
7. Arrange SCD sleeve under patient's leg according to leg position indicated on inner lining of sleeve. Correct leg position on inner lining.	☐	☐	_____
Back of patient's ankle should line up with ankle on inner lining of sleeve.	☐	☐	_____
Position back of patient's knee with popliteal opening.	☐	☐	_____
8. Wrap SCD sleeve securely around patient's leg.	☐	☐	_____
9. Verify fit of SCD sleeves by placing two fingers between patient's leg and sleeve. Check fit of SCD sleeve.	☐	☐	_____
10. Attach connector of SCD sleeve to plug on mechanical unit. Arrow on compressor lines up with arrow on plug from mechanical unit. Align arrows when connecting to mechanical unit.	☐	☐	_____
11. Turn mechanical unit on. Green light indicates that unit is functioning.	☐	☐	_____
12. Observe functioning of unit for one complete cycle.	☐	☐	_____
13. Reposition patient for comfort and perform hand hygiene.	☐	☐	_____
14. Remove compression stockings at least once per shift.	☐	☐	_____
15. Document the procedure.	☐	☐	_____

This page intentionally left blank

PROCEDURE 27-3

APPLYING ANTIEMBOLIC ELASTIC STOCKINGS

	S	U	Comments

1. Identify patient using two identifiers (i.e., name and birth date or name and account number, according to agency policy). ☐ ☐ _____

2. Observe for signs, symptoms, and condition of patient skin that contraindicate use of antiembolic elastic stockings. Signs and symptoms include:

   a. Dermatitis or open skin lesion ☐ ☐ _____

   b. Recent skin graft ☐ ☐ _____

   c. Decreased circulation in lower extremities as evidenced by cyanotic, cool extremities, gangrenous conditions affecting lower limb(s) ☐ ☐ _____

   Notify the nurse if any of these are present.

3. Assess and document condition of patient's skin and circulation to leg and foot (i.e.,presence of popliteal and pedal pulses, edema, and discoloration of skin; temperature; lesions; or abrasions) ☐ ☐ _____

4. Use tape measure to measure patient's legs to determine proper stocking size. ☐ ☐ _____

5. Explain procedure and reasons for applying stockings. ☐ ☐ _____

6. Perform hand hygiene. Provide hygiene to patient's lower extremities as needed. ☐ ☐ _____

7. Position patient in supine position. ☐ ☐ _____

8. Apply elastic stockings:

   a. Turn elastic stocking inside out up to heel. Place one hand into stocking,holding heel. Pull top of stocking with other hand inside out over foot of stocking. ☐ ☐ _____

   b. Place patient's toes into foot of elastics tocking, making sure that stocking is smooth. Place toes into foot of stocking. ☐ ☐ _____

   c. Slide remaining portion of stocking over patient's foot, being sure that toes are covered. Make sure that foot fits into toe and heel position of stocking. Slide heel of stocking over foot. ☐ ☐ _____

301

Procedures Checklists

	S	U	Comments

d. Slide top of stocking up over patient's calf until stocking is completely extended. Be sure that stocking is smooth and that no ridges or wrinkles are present, particularly behind knee. Slide stocking up leg until completely extended. ☐ ☐ _____

e. Instruct patient not to roll stockings partially down. ☐ ☐ _____

9. Reposition patient for comfort and perform hand hygiene. ☐ ☐ _____

10. Remove stockings at least once per shift. ☐ ☐ _____

11. Inspect stockings for wrinkles or constriction. ☐ ☐ _____

12. Inspect elastic stockings to determine that there are no wrinkles, rolls, or binding. ☐ ☐ _____

13. Observe circulatory status of lower extremities. ☐ ☐ _____

14. Observe color, temperature, and condition of skin. Palpate pedal pulses. ☐ ☐ _____

15. Observe patient's response to wearing antiembolic elastic stockings. ☐ ☐ _____

16. Document the procedure. ☐ ☐ _____

PROCEDURE 28-1

APPLYING HEAT APPLICATIONS

	S	U	Comments
1. Sanitize your hands.	☐	☐	_____
2. Explain the procedure to the patient and answer any questions.	☐	☐	_____
3. Ask the patient to remove all jewelry from the area to be treated.	☐	☐	_____
4. Place one or two towel layers over the area to be treated.	☐	☐	_____
5. Apply the commercial moist heat packs.	☐	☐	_____
6. Cover with the remaining portion of the towel.	☐	☐	_____
7. Advise the patient to leave the heat pack in place no longer than 20 to 30 minutes, off for the same amount of time, and then repeat if needed.	☐	☐	_____
8. Record the procedure in the patient's medical record.	☐	☐	_____

This page intentionally left blank

PROCEDURE 28-2

APPLYING COLD APPLICATIONS

	S	U	Comments
1. Sanitize your hands.	☐	☐	_____
2. Explain the procedure to the patient and answer any questions.	☐	☐	_____
3. Check the bag for leaks.	☐	☐	_____
4. Fill the bag with small cubes or chips of ice until it is about two-thirds full.	☐	☐	_____
5. Push down on the top of the bag to expel excess air and put on the cap or seal the plastic bag.	☐	☐	_____
6. Dry the outside of the bag and cover it with one or two towel layers.	☐	☐	_____
7. Help the patient position the ice bag on the injured area.	☐	☐	_____
8. Advise the patient to leave the ice bag in place for about 20 to 30 minutes or until the area feels numb, whichever comes first. (Leaving the ice in place for longer than 20 to 30 minutes may cause tissue damage.)	☐	☐	_____
9. Check the skin for color, feeling, and pain every 2-3 minutes after the first 10 minutes of therapy. (If the treated area becomes very painful, remains numb, or is pale or cyanotic, the ice bag should be removed and the nurse notified.)	☐	☐	_____
10. Record the procedure in the patient's medical record.	☐	☐	_____

This page intentionally left blank

PROCEDURE 29-1

APPLYING A BANDAGE

	S	U	Comments
1. Refer to the medical record, care plan, or Kardex for special interventions.	☐	☐	_____
2. Introduction yourself to the patient; include name and title or role.	☐	☐	_____
3. Identify patient by checking armband and requesting that patient state his/her name.	☐	☐	_____
4. Explain the procedure and the reason for the procedure in terms the patient is able to understand; give the patient time to ask questions. Advise the patient of any potential unpleasantness that will be experienced.	☐	☐	_____
5. Perform hand hygiene and don clean gloves according to agency policy and guidelines from the CDC and the Occupational Safety and Health Administration (OSHA).	☐	☐	_____
6. Assemble equipment and complete necessary charges.	☐	☐	_____
7. Prepare patient for intervention:			
a. Close door or pull privacy curtain.	☐	☐	_____
b. Raise bed to comfortable working height; lower side rail on side nearest you.	☐	☐	_____
c. Position and drape patient as necessary.	☐	☐	_____
8. Ensure that skin and dressing are clean and dry.	☐	☐	_____
9. Separate any adjacent skin surfaces.	☐	☐	_____
10. Align part to be bandaged, providing slight flexion as appropriate and not contraindicated.	☐	☐	_____
11. Apply bandage from distal to proximal part.	☐	☐	_____
12. Apply bandage with even distribution of pressure.			
a. For the circular bandage, see Table 29.2.	☐	☐	_____
b. For the spiral bandage, see Table 29.2.	☐	☐	_____
c. For the spiral-reverse bandage, see Table 29.2.	☐	☐	_____

	S	U	Comments

d. For the recurrent (stump) bandage, see Table 29.2. ☐ ☐ _____

e. For the figure-of-8 bandage, see Table 29.2. ☐ ☐ _____

f. Secure first bandage before applying additional rolls. Apply additional rolls without leaving any uncovered areas. ☐ ☐ _____

13. Assess tension of bandage and circulation of extremity. ☐ ☐ _____

14. During the procedure, promote patient involvement as possible. ☐ ☐ _____

15. Assess patient's tolerance, being alert for signs and symptoms of discomfort and fatigue. Inability to tolerate a procedure is described in the nursing notes. ☐ ☐ _____

16. On completion of procedure, assist patient to a position of comfort and place needed items within easy reach. Be certain patient has a means to call for assistance and knows how to use it. ☐ ☐ _____

17. Raise the side rails and lower the bed to the lowest position. ☐ ☐ _____

18. Remove gloves and all protective barriers, such as gown, goggles, and masks if worn. Store or remove and dispose of soiled supplies and equipment according to agency policy and guidelines from the CDC and OSHA. ☐ ☐ _____

19. Perform hand hygiene after patient contact and after removing gloves. ☐ ☐ _____

20. Document patient's response, expected or unexpected outcomes, and patient teaching. Specific notes for documentation are included in each procedure. ☐ ☐ _____

21. Report any unexpected outcomes immediately to the nurse. Specific notes for reporting are included in each procedure. ☐ ☐ _____

PROCEDURE 29-2

APPLYING A BINDER, ARM SLING, AND T-BINDER

	S	U	Comments

1. Refer to the medical record, care plan, or Kardex for special interventions. ☐ ☐ _____

2. Provide an introduction to the patient; include name and title or role. ☐ ☐ _____

3. Identify patient by checking armband and requesting that patient state his/her name. ☐ ☐ _____

4. Explain the procedure and the reason for the procedure in terms the patient is able to understand; give the patient time to ask questions. Advise the patient of any potential unpleasantness that will be experienced. ☐ ☐ _____

5. Perform hand hygiene and don clean gloves according to agency policy and guidelines from the CDC and the Occupational Safety and Health Administration (OSHA). ☐ ☐ _____

6. Assemble equipment. ☐ ☐ _____

7. Prepare patient for intervention:

   a. Close door or pull privacy curtain. ☐ ☐ _____

   b. Raise bed to comfortable working height; lower side rail on side nearest you. ☐ ☐ _____

   c. Position and drape patient as necessary. ☐ ☐ _____

8. Change dressing if appropriate; cleanse skin if needed. ☐ ☐ _____

9. Separate skin surfaces or pad bony prominences. ☐ ☐ _____

10. Apply binder:

    a. Triangular binder (sling):

       (1) Have patient flex arm at approximately 80-degree angle, depending on purpose of binder. ☐ ☐ _____

       (2) Place end of triangular binder over shoulder of the uninjured side, anterior to posterior. ☐ ☐ _____

       (3) Grasp other end of binder and bring it up and over injured arm to shoulder of injured arm. ☐ ☐ _____

309

	S	U	Comments

(4) Use square knot to tie two ends together at lateral area of neck on uninjured side. ☐ ☐ _____

(5) Support wrist well with binder; do not allow it to extend over end of binder. ☐ ☐ _____

(6) Fold third triangle end neatly around elbow and secure with safety pins. ☐ ☐ _____

b. T-binder:

(1) Using appropriate binder, place the waistband smoothly under patient's waist; patient should be positioned lying supine; tails should be under patient. ☐ ☐ _____

(2) Secure two ends of waistband together with safety pin. ☐ ☐ _____

(3) Single tail: bring the tail up between legs to secure dressing in place. Two tails: bring tails up one on each side of penis or large dressing. ☐ ☐ _____

(4) Bring tails under and over waistband; secure with safety pins. ☐ ☐ _____

c. Elastic abdominal binder:

(1) Center binder smoothly under appropriate part of patient. ☐ ☐ _____

(2) Close binder: Pull one end of binder over center of patient's abdomen while maintaining tension on that end of binder; pull opposite end of binder over center and secure with Velcro closure tabs, metal fasteners, or horizontally placed safety pins. ☐ ☐ _____

(3) Observe patient's respiratory status. ☐ ☐ _____

d. For postsurgical application of abdominal binders, proceed upward from bottom (except for a patient after cesarean delivery) to minimize pull on the suture line. ☐ ☐ _____

11. Note comfort level of patient. Smooth out binder to prevent wrinkles. Adjust binder as necessary. ☐ ☐ _____

12. During the procedure: Promote patient involvement as possible. ☐ ☐ _____

13. Assess patient's tolerance, being alert for signs and symptoms of discomfort and fatigue. Inability to tolerate a procedure is described in the nursing notes. ☐ ☐ _____

	S	U	Comments

14. Completion of procedure: Assist patient to a position of comfort and place needed items within easy reach. Be certain patient has a means to call for assistance and knows how to use it. ☐ ☐ _____

15. Raise the side rails and lower the bed to the lowest position. ☐ ☐ _____

16. Remove gloves and all protective barriers, such as gown, goggles, and masks if worn. Store or remove and dispose of soiled supplies and equipment according to agency policy and guidelines from the CDC and OSHA. ☐ ☐ _____

17. Perform hand hygiene after patient contact and after removing gloves. ☐ ☐ _____

18. Document patient's response, expected or unexpected outcomes, and patient teaching. Specific notes for documentation are included in each procedure. ☐ ☐ _____

19. Report any unexpected outcomes immediately to the nurse. Specific notes for reporting are included in each procedure. ☐ ☐ _____

20. Document:

   Time of application ☐ ☐ _____

   Type of binder ☐ ☐ _____

   Patient's response ☐ ☐ _____

This page intentionally left blank

PROCEDURE 34-1

ADMINISTERING A NEBULIZER TREATMENT

	S	U	Comments
1. Plug the nebulizer into a properly grounded electrical outlet.	☐	☐	_____
2. Introduce yourself and confirm the patient's identity.	☐	☐	_____
3. Explain the purpose of the treatment.	☐	☐	_____
4. Sanitize your hands.	☐	☐	_____
5. Measure the prescribed dose of drug into the nebulizer medication cup.	☐	☐	_____
6. Replace the top of the medication cup and connect it to the mouthpiece or face mask.	☐	☐	_____
7. Connect the disposable tubing to the nebulizer and the medication cup.	☐	☐	_____
8. The patient should be sitting upright to allow for total lung expansion.	☐	☐	_____
9. Turn on the nebulizer. If using a mask, position it comfortably but securely over the patient's mouth and nose.	☐	☐	_____
10. If using a mouthpiece, instruct the patient to hold it between the teeth with the lips pursed around the mouthpiece.	☐	☐	_____
11. Encourage the patient to take slow, deep breaths through the mouth and to hold each breath 2 to 3 seconds to allow the medicati onto disperse through the lungs.	☐	☐	_____
12. Continue the treatment until aerosol is no longer produced (approximately 10 minutes).	☐	☐	_____
CAUTION: If the patient is receiving a bronchodilator (albuterol), he or she may experience dizziness, tremors, or tachycardia. Continue the treatment unless otherwise notified by the nurse.			
13. Turn off the nebulizer.	☐	☐	_____
14. Encourage the patient to take several deep breaths and to cough loosened secretions into disposable tissues.	☐	☐	_____

	S	U	Comments

15. Dispose of the mouthpiece or mask and tubing in a biohazard container and instruct the patient also to dispose of the contaminated tissues in the biohazard container. ☐ ☐ _____

16. Sanitize your hands. ☐ ☐ _____

17. Record the nebulizer treatment; the patient's response, including the amount of coughing and whether coughing was productive or nonproductive; and any side effects of the medication. ☐ ☐ _____

PROCEDURE 35-1

CARE OF THE BODY AFTER DEATH

	S	U	Comments
1. Gather equipment.	☐	☐	_____
2. Wash hands.	☐	☐	_____
3. Don clean gloves.	☐	☐	_____
4. Close patient's eyes and mouth if needed.	☐	☐	_____
5. Remove all tubing and other devices from patient's body. [Some situations require that all tubing remain in the body (e.g., when an autopsy is scheduled). Know agency policy.]	☐	☐	_____
6. Place patient in supine position. Elevate the head. Do not place one hand on top of the other.	☐	☐	_____
7. Replace soiled dressings with clean ones.	☐	☐	_____
8. Bathe patient as necessary.	☐	☐	_____
9. Brush or comb hair.	☐	☐	_____
10. Apply clean gown.	☐	☐	_____
11. Care for valuables and personal belongings. If wedding band is to remain on the deceased, secure ring to finger with a small strip of tape over ring.	☐	☐	_____
12. Allow family to view body and remain in room. A sheet or light blanket placed over the body with only the head and upper shoulders exposed maintains dignity and respect for the deceased. Remove unneeded equipment from the room. Provide soft lighting and offer chairs.	☐	☐	_____
13. After the family has left the room, attach special label if patient had a contagious disease.	☐	☐	_____
14. Close door to room.	☐	☐	_____
15. Await arrival of ambulance or transfer to morgue. (Some agencies use a shroud to enclose the body before transfer to the morgue.)	☐	☐	_____
16. Document procedure and disposition of patient's body and of belongings and valuables.	☐	☐	_____

This page intentionally left blank

Practice Exam

1. Karen is preparing to transfer a patient from the bed to a chair. What should Karen do prior to transferring the patient?
   1. Alert the nurse.
   2. Discontinue IV therapy.
   3. Check the area for clutter or rugs.
   4. Have the patient wear closed-toed shoes.

2. Which patient is at greater risk for orthostatic hypotension?
   1. patient taking insulin
   2. older patients with altered sensory perception
   3. patient taking medication to raise his blood pressure
   4. patient taking medication to lower his blood pressure

3. Which intervention prevents complications of immobility?
   1. a high-fiber diet
   2. limited ambulation
   3. adequate fluid intake
   4. reposition at least every 4 hours

4. Which position is appropriate for patients with a cardiac or respiratory condition?
   1. orthopneic
   2. semi-Fowler's
   3. Trendelenburg's
   4. dorsal recumbent

5. The patient care technician's first response in an active shooter situation is:
   1. remain calm.
   2. seek a place to hide.
   3. develop a plan to fight back.
   4. contact security and the police.

6. What is the rationale for enlisting the help of a coworker when moving a patient?
   1. increases stability
   2. keeps workload to a minimum
   3. divides the workload by 50%
   4. reduces risk of injury to the patient

7. The patient care technician is caring for an older patient who has been determined to be at risk for falls. On several occasions, the patient has attempted to get out of bed without requesting assistance. Which is appropriate to alert the patient care technician if this patient attempts to get out of bed again?
   1. locked bedrails
   2. restraints
   3. call button
   4. weight-sensitive alarm

8. The patient care technician should ensure that the call light or signal system is working and accessible to promote:
   1. a safe environment.
   2. good communication.
   3. good customer service.
   4. compliance with hospital regulations.

9. Carla, the patient care technician, is caring for a patient who just who had a surgical procedure for which he received narcotics for analgesia. What should Carla do when the patient awakens and asks to go to the restroom?
   1. Check blood pressure.
   2. Place the patient in a wheelchair.
   3. Assist the patient when getting out of bed.
   4. Confirm with the nurse that the patient can get out of bed.

10. The wound caused by stepping on a nail is an example of a(n):
    1. contusion.
    2. abrasion.
    3. avulsion.
    4. puncture.

11. A skinned knee or rug burn is an example of a(n):
    1. contusion.
    2. abrasion.
    3. avulsion.
    4. puncture.

12. Which is an example of a health promotion strategy?
    1. checking glucose levels before meals
    2. monitoring blood pressure
    3. finishing all medication as prescribed
    4. making dietary changes to prevent elevated cholesterol

13. Health disparities may be based on: *(Select all that apply.)*
    1. income.
    2. disability.
    3. religion.
    4. race.
    5. sexual orientation.

14. Alex is trying to take vital signs for a patient who has just arrived in the health clinic during a busy time. The patient has anxiety about being sick. Alex, very cognizant of the packed waiting room, ignores the patient's concerns and proceeds to take her blood pressure. The patient, startled, squeals as the blood pressure cuff tightens. Alex scolds, "You have to remain still!" Which communication style best describes Alex's response in this situation?
    1. nonverbal communication
    2. one-way communication
    3. aggressive communication
    4. assertive communication

15. The nursing student leaves a copy of a patient's Kardex on a bedside table. A visitor finds the copy and reads it. What should the student do?
    1. Take the Kardex out of the patient's room and immediately shred it.
    2. Apologize to the visitor and patient and explain the information on the Kardex.
    3. Obtain the copy of the Kardex and check for patient identifiers.
    4. Retrieve the Kardex, contact instructor, and complete an incident report.

16. Which skills are included in the role of a patient care technician? *(Select all that apply.)*
    1. diagnosing conditions
    2. oxygen delivery
    3. phlebotomy
    4. intravenous therapy
    5. electrocardiogram

17. Which should the patient care technician avoid in the workplace? *(Select all that apply.)*
    1. earrings
    2. tennis shoes
    3. tongue piercings
    4. makeup
    5. long fingernails

18. The patient asks the patient care technician her opinion regarding the physician's prescribed course of treatment. The technician suggests alternate treatment options for the patient to consider. The technician has just:
    1. taken initiative.
    2. practiced medicine without a license.
    3. shown credibility.
    4. been a team player.

19. A person is considered to have a substance abuse problem if which is true?
    1. increased impulsiveness or recklessness
    2. continued social or interpersonal problems
    3. mood swings
    4. use that results in legal problems

20. A terminally ill patient wants to discontinue treatment. The treatment has made the patient extremely ill and the patient believes continuing treatment would adversely impact her quality of life. The patient care technician thinks the clinical staff should support and advocate in support of this patient's decision. This is an example of:
    1. ethics.
    2. beneficence.
    3. duty of care.
    4. nonmaleficence.

21. The patient care technician makes numerous social media posts spreading unfounded rumors accusing a coworker of making mistakes that caused harm to patients. This is known as:
    1. assault.
    2. libel.
    3. slander.
    4. defamation.

22. A person or animal that does not become ill but harbors and spreads an organism that causes disease in others is called a:
    1. spore.
    2. vector.
    3. host.
    4. fomite.

23. The patient care technician understands that infections result from a specific chain of events. Which practice(s) stop(s) or slow(s) the chain of infection events? *(Select all that apply.)*
    1. handwashing
    2. sterilizing surgical instruments
    3. wearing protective equipment
    4. private rooms for all patients with communicable diseases
    5. workers with draining lesions should avoid direct patient care

24. Which is/are invasive technique(s)? *(Select all that apply.)*
    1. acupuncture
    2. chiropractic manipulation
    3. an epidural
    4. tissue palpitation
    5. neurosurgical procedures

25. The nurse is caring for a patient who has arthritis. Which nonpharmacologic intervention is likely to be used for the pain?
    1. massage
    2. heat or cold application
    3. progressive muscle relaxation
    4. transcutaneous electric nerve stimulation

26. Which physical examination method ranges from focusing on the patient's general appearance to more detailed observations?
    1. auscultation
    2. palpation
    3. mensuration
    4. manipulation

27. A sweet, fruity-smelling breath can be indicative of which condition?
    1. lung disease
    2. renal disease
    3. liver disease
    4. dehydration

28. Which rhythm is shown in the illustration below?
    1. Sinus tachycardia
    2. Sinus bradycardia
    3. Ventricular tachycardia
    4. Ventricular fibrillation

29. Which rhythm is shown in the illustration below?
    1. Sinus tachycardia
    2. Normal sinus rhythm
    3. Ventricular tachycardia
    4. Ventricular fibrillation

30. A patient who is anxious or in pain may have an increase in the pulse rate, which is called:
    1. tachycardia.
    2. a pulse deficit.
    3. an intermittent pulse.
    4. sinus arrhythmia.

31. Which is an anthropometric measurement? *(Select all that apply.)*
    1. pulse
    2. temperature
    3. respiratory rate
    4. head and chest circumference

32. The patient care technician is initiating admission procedures for a patient being admitted through the emergency department. Which is the priority?
    1. starting treatment
    2. orienting the patient to his room
    3. getting the patient to the nursing unit
    4. obtaining vital information from the patient

33. Drugs enter the body through which of the following enteral routes: *(Select all that apply.)*
    1. topical
    2. lozenges
    3. suspensions
    4. Instillation
    5. suppositories

34. The patient care technician knows that which patients are at risk for urine elimination problems?
    1. Older patients
    2. Severely obese patients
    3. Patients with hemorrhoids
    4. Patients recovering from prostate surgery

35. Which is an accurate principle of medical asepsis?
    1. Remove all unnecessary equipment.
    2. Place soiled linen in the biohazard bag.
    3. Fan linen in the air before making the bed.
    4. Place soiled linen on the floor and place in the hamper after making the bed with clean linen.

36. A patient is receiving transtracheal oxygen delivery. During the patient's inspection of the transtracheal tract opening, the patient notices small amounts of clear exudate. What should the patient care technician do?
    1. Clean the area.
    2. Inform the patient that this is normal.
    3. Discontinue treatment.
    4. Inform the nurse immediately.

37. Which is a side effect of regular enema use?
    1. dehydration
    2. diarrhea
    3. constipation
    4. infection

38. Which is the most appropriate action for the patient care technician dressing a patient?
    1. Ensure that the patient wears a belt.
    2. Select the patient's clothing for the day.
    3. Change the patient's gown when the IV solution container is changed.
    4. Discontinue the IV, if the patient has one, before changing the patient's gown.

39. Which is/are component(s) of the physical examination of urine? *(Select all that apply.)*
    1. pH
    2. foam
    3. volume
    4. ketones
    5. appearance

40. Routine adult venipuncture requires a _____-gauge needle.
    1. 16
    2. 23
    3. 20- to 21
    4. 21- to 22

41. Which surgical procedure uses extreme cold to destroy tissues such as warts and skin lesions?
    1. cryosurgery
    2. microsurgery
    3. electrosurgery
    4. endoscopic surgery

42. A heat application is likely to be used for:
    1. a sprain.
    2. a fracture.
    3. back pain.
    4. a nosebleed.

43. Which group has the highest incidence of keloid formation?
    1. women
    2. diabetics
    3. older adults
    4. African-Americans

44. Which observation of the newborn's bowel function should be reported to the health care provider?
    1. Initial stool is black-green with a sticky consistency.
    2. Stool contains strands of lanugo, mucus, and vernix.
    3. No stool is passed 24 hours after birth.
    4. Newborn appears to be straining when passing stool.

45. Which is/are risk factor(s) for cognitive decline? *(Select all that apply.)*
    1. kidney disease
    2. hypertension
    3. lead exposure
    4. poor nutrition
    5. lack of social interaction

46. The patient care technician is speaking with the parent of a 16-year-old girl who has diabetes. The mother says that her daughter has been refusing to monitor her glucose levels or take her medicine. Usually bubbly and social, her daughter has taken to staying in bed and has become increasingly reclusive. The mother thought that her daughter was starting to cheer up when she invited her friends over but her hopes were dashed when she realized that her daughter had only invited them over to distribute many of her belongings. The daughter is exhibiting signs of:
    1. anxiety.
    2. stress.
    3. drug abuse.
    4. suicide risk.

47. Which of the following is a common problem for older adults?
    1. Obesity
    2. Incontinence
    3. Depression
    4. Polypharmacy

48. The patient is a large man who needs assistance to move and transfer to a wheelchair. His wife, the caregiver, is a relatively small woman. Who would be contacted first to address this problem?
    1. interdisciplinary team
    2. hospice aide
    3. physical therapist
    4. nurse coordinator

49. The patient care technician overhears a colleague criticizing a patient who is a Jehovah's Witness and is declining a blood transfusion. The colleague declares, "I'm so glad I'm not a Jehovah's Witness. Christians don't believe that crazy stuff! Somebody needs to talk some sense into her and bring her over to this side!" The colleague's attitude reflects:
    1. bigotry.
    2. ethnocentrism.
    3. insufficient health literacy.
    4. lack of culturally competent care.

50. Driver's education, water safety training, education about _____, and drug education are necessary to inform adolescents of the risks and dangers inherent in these activities.
    1. fitness
    2. nutrition
    3. bullying
    4. safe sex practices